NATIONAL ACADEMIES *Sciences Engineering Medicine*

NATIONAL ACADEMIES PRESS
Washington, DC

Defining and Evaluating In-Home Drug Disposal Systems for Opioid Analgesics

Theresa Wizemann, Kyle Cavagnini, and Carolyn Shore, *Rapporteurs*

Forum on Drug Discovery, Development, and Translation

Board on Health Sciences Policy

Health and Medicine Division

Proceedings of a Workshop

NATIONAL ACADEMIES PRESS 500 Fifth Street, NW Washington, DC 20001

This activity was supported by Amgen Inc.; Association of American Medical Colleges; AstraZeneca; Biogen; Burroughs Wellcome Fund (Award No. 1023129); Critical Path Institute; Eli Lilly and Company; FasterCures, Milken Institute; Food and Drug Administration (Grant No. 1R13FD007302-01); Foundation for the National Institutes of Health; Friends of Cancer Research; Johnson & Johnson; Medable, Inc.; Merck & Co., Inc. (Award No. MRLCPO-23-166623); National Institutes of Health (Contract No. HHSN263201800029I; Task Order No. HHSN26300007): National Cancer Institute, National Institute of Allergy and Infectious Diseases, National Institute of Mental Health, National Institute of Neurological Disorders and Stroke, Office of Science Policy; *New England Journal of Medicine*; and Sanofi (Contract No. 77646387). Any opinions, findings, conclusions, or recommendations expressed in this publication do not necessarily reflect the views of any organization or agency that provided support for the project.

International Standard Book Number-13: 978-0-309-71434-1
International Standard Book Number-10: 0-309-71434-6
Digital Object Identifier: https://doi.org/10.17226/27436

This publication is available from the National Academies Press, 500 Fifth Street, NW, Keck 360, Washington, DC 20001; (800) 624-6242 or (202) 334-3313; http://www.nap.edu.

Copyright 2024 by the National Academy of Sciences. National Academies of Sciences, Engineering, and Medicine and National Academies Press and the graphical logos for each are all trademarks of the National Academy of Sciences. All rights reserved.

Printed in the United States of America.

Suggested citation: National Academies of Sciences, Engineering, and Medicine. 2024. *Defining and evaluating in-home drug disposal systems for opioid analgesics: Proceedings of a workshop*. Washington, DC: The National Academies Press. https://doi.org/10.17226/27436.

The **National Academy of Sciences** was established in 1863 by an Act of Congress, signed by President Lincoln, as a private, nongovernmental institution to advise the nation on issues related to science and technology. Members are elected by their peers for outstanding contributions to research. Dr. Marcia McNutt is president.

The **National Academy of Engineering** was established in 1964 under the charter of the National Academy of Sciences to bring the practices of engineering to advising the nation. Members are elected by their peers for extraordinary contributions to engineering. Dr. John L. Anderson is president.

The **National Academy of Medicine** (formerly the Institute of Medicine) was established in 1970 under the charter of the National Academy of Sciences to advise the nation on medical and health issues. Members are elected by their peers for distinguished contributions to medicine and health. Dr. Victor J. Dzau is president.

The three Academies work together as the **National Academies of Sciences, Engineering, and Medicine** to provide independent, objective analysis and advice to the nation and conduct other activities to solve complex problems and inform public policy decisions. The National Academies also encourage education and research, recognize outstanding contributions to knowledge, and increase public understanding in matters of science, engineering, and medicine.

Learn more about the National Academies of Sciences, Engineering, and Medicine at **www.nationalacademies.org**.

Consensus Study Reports published by the National Academies of Sciences, Engineering, and Medicine document the evidence-based consensus on the study's statement of task by an authoring committee of experts. Reports typically include findings, conclusions, and recommendations based on information gathered by the committee and the committee's deliberations. Each report has been subjected to a rigorous and independent peer-review process and it represents the position of the National Academies on the statement of task.

Proceedings published by the National Academies of Sciences, Engineering, and Medicine chronicle the presentations and discussions at a workshop, symposium, or other event convened by the National Academies. The statements and opinions contained in proceedings are those of the participants and are not endorsed by other participants, the planning committee, or the National Academies.

Rapid Expert Consultations published by the National Academies of Sciences, Engineering, and Medicine are authored by subject-matter experts on narrowly focused topics that can be supported by a body of evidence. The discussions contained in rapid expert consultations are considered those of the authors and do not contain policy recommendations. Rapid expert consultations are reviewed by the institution before release.

For information about other products and activities of the National Academies, please visit www.nationalacademies.org/about/whatwedo.

PLANNING COMMITTEE ON DEFINING AND EVALUATING IN-HOME DRUG DISPOSAL SYSTEMS FOR OPIOID ANALGESICS[1]

ELIZABETH McGINTY (*Co-Chair*), Chief, Division of Health Policy and Economics, and Professor, Department of Population Health Sciences, Weill Cornell Medicine
ALASTAIR J. J. WOOD (*Co-Chair*), Professor of Medicine Emeritus, Vanderbilt University School of Medicine
MARK C. BICKET, Assistant Professor, Director, Pain & Opioid Research, Department of Anesthesiology, Institute for Healthcare Policy and Innovation, University of Michigan Medical School
IRENE Z. CHAN, Deputy Director, Office of Medication Error Prevention and Risk Management, Center for Drug Evaluation and Research, Food and Drug Administration
RUCHI M. FITZGERALD, Assistant Professor, Rush University; Service Chief of Inpatient Addiction Medicine, PCC Community Wellness Center
LEWIS GROSSMAN, Ann Loeb Bronfman Professor of Law, American University Washington College of Law
STEPHEN W. HOAG, Professor of Pharmaceutical Sciences, University of Maryland Baltimore School of Pharmacy
ROBERT MORONES, Injury Prevention Specialist, Indian Health Service (Phoenix Area), U.S. Department of Health and Human Services
THOMAS PRISINZANO, Professor and Chair, Pharmaceutical Sciences Department, University of Kentucky College of Pharmacy
JESSICA YOUNG, Chief, Recycling and Generator Branch, Environmental Protection Agency
PATRICIA J. ZETTLER, Associate Professor, The Ohio State University Moritz College of Law

Staff

CAROLYN SHORE, Director, Forum on Drug Discovery, Development, and Translation
KYLE CAVAGNINI, Associate Program Officer
MAYA THIRKILL, Associate Program Officer (*until May 2023*)
NOAH ONTJES, Research Associate

---

[1] The National Academies of Sciences, Engineering, and Medicine's planning committees are solely responsible for organizing the workshop, identifying topics, and choosing speakers. The responsibility for the published Proceedings of a Workshop rests with the workshop rapporteurs and the institution.

MELVIN JOPPY, Senior Program Assistant
CLARE STROUD, Senior Director, Board on Health Sciences Policy

Consultant

THERESA WIZEMANN, Science Writer

FORUM ON DRUG DISCOVERY, DEVELOPMENT, AND TRANSLATION[1]

GREGORY SIMON (*Co-Chair*), Kaiser Permanente Washington Health Research Institute and University of Washington
ANN TAYLOR (*Co-Chair*), Retired
BARBARA E. BIERER, Harvard Medical School; Brigham and Women's Hospital
LINDA BRADY, National Institute of Mental Health, NIH
JOHN BUSE, University of North Carolina at Chapel Hill School of Medicine
LUTHER T. CLARK, Merck & Co., Inc.
BARRY S. COLLER, The Rockefeller University
TAMMY R.L. COLLINS, Burroughs Wellcome Fund
THOMAS CURRAN, Children's Mercy, Kansas City
RICHARD DAVEY, National Institute of Allergy and Infectious Diseases, NIH
KATHERINE DAWSON, Biogen
JAMES H. DOROSHOW, National Cancer Institute, NIH
JEFFREY M. DRAZEN, *New England Journal of Medicine*
STEVEN K. GALSON, Retired
CARLOS O. GARNER, Eli Lilly and Company
SALLY L. HODDER, West Virginia University
TESHEIA JOHNSON, Yale School of Medicine
LYRIC JORGENSON, Office of Science Policy, NIH
ESTHER KROFAH, FasterCures, Milken Institute
LISA M. LaVANGE, University of North Carolina
ARAN MAREE, Johnson & Johnson
CRISTIAN MASSACESI, AstraZeneca
ROSS McKINNEY, JR., Association of American Medical Colleges
JOSEPH P. MENETSKI, Foundation for the National Institutes of Health
ANAEZE C. OFFODILE II, University of Texas MD Anderson Cancer Center
SALLY OKUN, Clinical Trials Transformation Initiative
ARTI RAI, Duke University School of Law
KLAUS ROMERO, Critical Path Institute
JONI RUTTER, National Center for Advancing Translational Sciences, NIH

---

[1] The National Academies of Sciences, Engineering, and Medicine's forums and roundtables do not issue, review, or approve individual documents. The responsibility for the published Proceedings of a Workshop rests with the workshop rapporteurs and the institution.

SUSAN SCHAEFFER, The Patients' Academy for Research Advocacy
ANANTHA SHEKHAR, University of Pittsburgh School of Medicine
ELLEN V. SIGAL, Friends of Cancer Research
MARK TAISEY, Amgen Inc.
AMIR TAMIZ, National Institute of Neurological Disorders and Stroke, NIH
PAMELA TENAERTS, Medable, Inc.
MAJID VAKILYNEJAD, Takeda
JONATHAN WATANABE, University of California, Irvine, School of Pharmacy and Pharmaceutical Sciences
ALASTAIR WOOD, Vanderbilt University School of Medicine
CRIS WOOLSTON, Sanofi
JOSEPH C. WU, Stanford University School of Medicine

Forum Staff

CAROLYN SHORE, Forum Director
KYLE CAVAGNINI, Associate Program Officer
BRITTANY HSIAO, Associate Program Officer (*as of September 2023*)
MAYA THIRKILL, Associate Program Officer (*until April 2023*)
NOAH ONTJES, Research Associate
MELVIN JOPPY, Senior Program Assistant
CLARE STROUD, Senior Director, Board on Health Sciences Policy

Reviewers

This Proceedings of a Workshop was reviewed in draft form by individuals chosen for their diverse perspectives and technical expertise. The purpose of this independent review is to provide candid and critical comments that will assist the National Academies of Sciences, Engineering, and Medicine in making each published proceedings as sound as possible and to ensure that it meets the institutional standards for quality, objectivity, evidence, and responsiveness to the charge. The review comments and draft manuscript remain confidential to protect the integrity of the process.

We thank the following individuals for their review of this proceedings:

MARK BICKET, University of Michigan Medical School
STEPHANIE Y. CRAWFORD, University of Illinois Chicago
ANDREA TSATOKE, Indian Health Service

Although the reviewers listed above provided many constructive comments and suggestions, they were not asked to endorse the content of the proceedings nor did they see the final draft before its release. The review of this proceedings was overseen by **ELI Y. ADASHI,** Brown University. He was responsible for making certain that an independent examination of this proceedings was carried out in accordance with standards of the National Academies and that all review comments were carefully considered. Responsibility for the final content rests entirely with the rapporteurs and the National Academies.

Acknowledgments

Support from the sponsors of the Forum on Drug Discovery, Development, and Translation is crucial to support this and other work of the National Academies of Sciences, Engineering, and Medicine (the National Academies).

The National Academies' staff wish to express their gratitude to the speakers whose presentations helped inform workshop discussions on defining and evaluating in-home drug disposal systems and their use; to the members of the planning committee for their work in developing the workshop agenda and shaping the discussions; and to additional National Academies' staff, without whom this workshop and the accounting thereof would not have been possible: Christie Bell, Samantha Chao, Robert Day, Alexandra Molina, Rebekah Hanover Pettit, Marguerite Romatelli, Lauren Shern, and Taryn Young.

Contents

ACRONYMS AND ABBREVIATIONS   xvii

1 INTRODUCTION   1
   The FDA Overdose Prevention Framework, 3
   Organization of the Proceedings, 5

2 LIFE CYCLE OF PRESCRIBED OPIOIDS   7
   Non-Medical Use, 8
   Diversion and Misuse, 8
   Drug Disposal, 9
   Intervention Points, 10

3 ENVISIONING DISPOSAL SYSTEMS TO REMOVE OPIOIDS
   FROM THE HOME   11
   Design and Its Relation to Human Behavior, 12
   Designing Usable In-Home Opioid Disposal Systems, 14

4 THE ROLE OF IN-HOME OPIOID DISPOSAL   21
   Facilitating In-Home Disposal of Opioid Analgesics, 22
   Considering the Roles of In-Home Disposal, 25

5 RISK EVALUATION AND MITIGATION STRATEGY (REMS)   33
   REMS Format and Content, 35
   REMS Modification, 35

    Overlapping Statutory Authorities for Controlled
       Substances, 36
    SUPPORT Act Provisions, 36
    Practical Considerations, 37

6 REGULATORY LANDSCAPE FOR HOUSEHOLD OPIOID
   DISPOSAL   39
   Product Stewardship, 40
   Perspectives on Regulatory Authority, 43

7 SCIENTIFIC CONSIDERATIONS FOR IN-HOME OPIOID
   DISPOSAL   49
   Assessing Utility and Performance, 50
   Scientific Considerations, 55

8 REAL-WORLD IMPLEMENTATION AND USE OF IN-
   HOME OPIOID DISPOSAL SYSTEMS   61
   Opportunities and Barriers for the Disposal of Unused
      Opioids, 62
   Real-World Experience, 65

9 REFLECTIONS ON THE DESIGN AND IMPLEMENTATION
   OF IN-HOME OPIOID DISPOSAL SYSTEMS   73
   Participant Reflections, 75

REFERENCES   83

APPENDIXES

A WORKSHOP AGENDA   85
B BIOGRAPHICAL SKETCHES OF THE WORKSHOP
    PLANNING COMMITTEE MEMBERS, SPEAKERS,
    AND PANELISTS   95

Boxes and Figures

BOXES

1-1 Workshop Statement of Task, 2

7-1 Key Performance Questions for Disposal Systems Assessed in the 2019 Report on In-Home Disposal Systems, 51

FIGURES

2-1 How misused prescription pain relievers are obtained, 9

5-1 Risk-based drug approval continuum, 34

6-1 Timeline of pharmaceuticals stewardship laws, 41

Acronyms and Abbreviations

CDC	Centers for Disease Control and Prevention
CDER	Center for Drug Evaluation and Research (FDA)
DEA	Drug Enforcement Administration
EHR	electronic health record
EPA	Environmental Protection Agency
EPR	extended producer responsibility
ETASU	elements to assure safe use
FDA	Food and Drug Administration
HHS	U.S. Department of Health and Human Services
HUB	Healthcare, Universal Design, and Biomechanics
ICD	*International Classification of Diseases*
IHS	Indian Health Service
NACDS	National Association of Chain Drug Stores
NIDA	National Institute on Drug Abuse (National Institutes of Health)
NPI	national provider identifier
ONDCP	White House Office of National Drug Control Policy
OPEN	Opioid Prescribing Engagement Network

OTC	over the counter
PSI	Product Stewardship Institute
RCRA	Resource Conservation and Recovery Act
RCT	randomized controlled trial
REMS	risk evaluation and mitigation strategy
SAFE	Stop the Addiction Fatality Epidemic
SUPPORT Act	Substance Use-Disorder Prevention that Promotes Opioid Recovery and Treatment for Patients and Communities Act of 2018
USPS	United States Postal Service
VA	U.S. Department of Veterans Affairs

1

Introduction[1]

The Substance Use-Disorder Prevention that Promotes Opioid Recovery and Treatment (SUPPORT) for Patients and Communities Act of 2018 (Public Law 115-271) gave the Food and Drug Administration (FDA) authority to require that drug manufacturers provide a safe drug disposal system for certain drugs that pose a serious risk of non-medical use or overdose, if FDA determines that the disposal system could mitigate that risk. The requirement to make in-home disposal systems available to patients would be implemented under a risk evaluation and mitigation strategy (REMS). On June 26–27, 2023, the Forum on Drug Discovery, Development, and Translation of the National Academies of Sciences, Engineering, and Medicine (the National Academies) hosted a public workshop as a venue for stakeholders to examine the development and use of in-home drug disposal systems, with a focus on removing unused opioid analgesics from the home. The National Academies appointed an ad-hoc planning committee to address the statement of task (Box 1-1).

Alastair Wood, professor of medicine emeritus at Vanderbilt University School of Medicine, said the workshop agenda was designed to

---

[1] This workshop was organized by an independent planning committee whose role was limited to identification of topics and speakers. This Proceedings of a Workshop was prepared by the rapporteurs as a factual summary of the presentations and discussions that took place at the workshop. Statements, recommendations, and opinions expressed are those of individual presenters and participants and are not endorsed or verified by the National Academies of Sciences, Engineering, and Medicine, and they should not be construed as reflecting any group consensus.

> **BOX 1-1**
> **Workshop Statement of Task**
>
> A planning committee of the National Academies of Sciences, Engineering, and Medicine will organize a public workshop on the development and use of in-home drug disposal systems with a focus on removing unused opioid analgesics from the home. The public workshop will feature invited presentations and discussions to:
>
> - Explore the types of in-home drug disposal options, other than mail-back envelopes, that could be used to remove unused opioid analgesics from the home.
> - Examine the current landscape of laws and regulations that apply to in-home opioid disposal systems.
> - Discuss scientific, behavioral, health equity, and policy considerations for assessing the safety, use, and effectiveness of in-home opioid disposal systems, including the following questions:
>   - What is known/unknown about the methods (e.g., sequestration, adsorption, absorption) used in in-home disposal systems for rendering opioids unavailable for non-medical use, assuming the product is used as intended?
>   - What approaches/methodologies are needed to evaluate the safe and correct use of in-home opioid disposal systems in real-world settings?
>   - How could person-centered design inform the development and use of in-home opioid disposal systems?
> - Consider potential strategies for encouraging and assessing the development and use of in-home opioid disposal systems that support the public health goal of mitigating the risk of non-medical use or overdose associated with opioids.
>
> The planning committee will organize the workshop, develop the agenda, select and invite speakers and discussants, and moderate or identify moderators for the discussions. A proceedings of the presentations and discussions at the workshop will be prepared by a designated rapporteur in accordance with institutional guidelines.

gather information on topics such as how well in-home disposal systems work to remove opioids from the home; the impact of in-home disposal systems on reducing opioid misuse; barriers and facilitators impacting whether people will actually use a provided in-home disposal system; and the safety of disposal systems themselves, including user safety when used as intended or otherwise, as well as safety risks for those attempting to recover drugs that have been disposed of in a system. The workshop also included discussions of the types of evidence that FDA might need if the REMS for opioid analgesics were to be expanded to include in-home opioid disposal systems (e.g., evidence of efficacy, safety, practicality, user acceptability, environmental impact).

THE FDA OVERDOSE PREVENTION FRAMEWORK

Marta Sokolowska, deputy center director for substance use and behavioral health at the FDA Center for Drug Evaluation and Research (CDER), provided a brief overview of FDA's Overdose Prevention framework and the agency's authority to regulate in-home opioid disposal systems.

Provisional data from the Centers for Disease Control and Prevention (CDC) indicate there were around 110,000 drug overdose deaths in the United States in 2022, the majority of which involved opioids, Sokolowska said. Furthermore, "the 2021 National Survey on Drug Use and Health estimates that 8.7 million people aged 12 and older misused prescription pain relievers in 2021," she said. A recent study of fatal poisonings in young children identified opioids as the most common cause (Gaw et al., 2023). Despite efforts to promote more appropriate prescribing, a recent systematic review found that 50 to 70 percent of opioid tablets prescribed for postsurgical pain management were not used (Mallama et al., 2022).

The National Drug Control Strategy issued by the White House Office of National Drug Control Policy (ONDCP) in 2022 calls for consistent guidance on the safe disposal of unused prescription drugs. To this end, FDA is collaborating with the United States Postal Service (USPS), the Drug Enforcement Administration (DEA), the Environmental Protection Agency (EPA), CDC, and other governmental agencies on this issue. "It is our shared responsibility to address the significant risk of non-medical use, accidental exposure, overdose, and death associated with unused opioids in patients' homes," Sokolowska said.

In alignment with the National Drug Control Strategy and the U.S. Department of Health and Human Services (HHS) Overdose Prevention Strategy, FDA launched its Overdose Prevention Framework in 2022. The framework prioritizes "primary prevention, harm reduction, providing evidence-based treatment for substance use disorders, and supporting safe drug supply," Sokolowska said, and is "guided by the same four crosscutting principles as the HHS strategy: equity; data and evidence; coordination, collaboration, and integration; and reducing stigma."

Under the primary prevention priority area, FDA is working to "eliminate unnecessary initial prescription exposure and inappropriate prolonged prescribing" of opioid medications, Sokolowska said. Initiatives have included product label changes that promote safer use and supporting the development of clinical practice guidelines for safer pain management prescribing.

The agency is also focused on identifying approaches for the safe removal of unused opioids from patient homes as a primary prevention strategy using its authority under the 2018 SUPPORT Act. Current options for disposing of unused opioids include collection kiosks and DEA's National Prescription Drug Take Back Days, which Sokolowska noted require patients to store unused opioids in the home until a local take-back day or until they can travel to a kiosk. There are also in-home disposal options, such as "flushing; mixing opioids with unpalatable substances and disposing them in trash; using commercially available in-home disposal systems and disposing them in trash; and having patients put unused opioids in mail-back envelopes that are transported to a facility for incineration," she continued.

Sokolowska elaborated on the mail-back option. Following a call for public comment on this issue in April 2022, FDA is modifying the current Opioid Analgesic REMS to require manufacturers of opioids to make prepaid mail-back envelopes available to outpatient dispensers (e.g., retail pharmacies) to provide to patients when dispensing prescribed opioids. Manufacturers must also develop patient education materials on safe disposal of opioids for dispensers to provide to patients.

While moving forward with the prepaid mail-back envelope strategy, FDA is also considering public feedback regarding the need for additional in-home disposal options. For example, Sokolowska said many patients and health care providers reported a preference for in-home disposal systems that can be discarded in household trash because they are "easier to use, less expensive, or less subject to diversion." Feedback from retail pharmacists indicates that "patients are familiar with using in-home disposal systems and appreciate receiving these with their medications," she said. There were also concerns raised by those in rural and Tribal communities that limited access to postal services made the use of mail-back envelopes less practical. She added that data in the literature suggest that counseling patients about opioid disposal and making in-home disposal options available promote disposal (Butler et al., 2021).

Under the authority provided by the SUPPORT Act, FDA is considering "where and under what circumstances to require other home disposal systems ... be provided to patients dispensed opioid analgesics," Sokolowska said. She explained that the SUPPORT Act, as passed in 2018, required that these in-home disposal systems render the medications "non-retrievable," a standard that refers to a controlled substance being rendered unusable for all practical purposes by means of irreversible physical or chemical changes to a substance (21 CFR § 1300.05). The non-retrievable requirement was "explicitly removed" from the SUPPORT Act in the Consolidated Appropriations Act of 2023.

Sokolowska emphasized that the agency has not made a decision on whether to expand the Opioid Analgesic REMS to include in-home disposal systems. FDA is seeking public input on this matter through a call for comments in the Federal Register.[2] The agency is eager to hear from patients and health care providers regarding "beliefs and perceptions around in-home disposal products, including those related to ease of use and environmental impact, as well as beliefs and perceptions that can impact willingness to use these products," she said.

ORGANIZATION OF THE PROCEEDINGS

This Proceedings of a Workshop summarizes the presentations and discussions that took place during the public workshop held on June 26 and 27, 2023. Chapter 2 presents an overview of the life cycle of prescribed opioids, from the prescribing encounter to after the patient has completed or stopped treatment, including the potential for non-medical use, diversion, and misuse along the pathway. Chapter 3 discusses characteristics of usable in-home opioid disposal systems, barriers to their implementation and use, and health equity considerations in the development of in-home disposal systems. Chapter 4 considers the role of an ideal in-home opioid disposal system in mitigating the risk of misuse or overdose of unused prescription opioids. An overview of the legal and practical aspects of REMS is provided in Chapter 5, followed by panelist perspectives on the current laws and regulations relevant to in-home drug disposal systems in Chapter 6. Chapter 7 considers the ideal characteristics of an in-home drug disposal system from mechanistic, safety, and environmental perspectives, and approaches for assessing the environmental impact of such systems. In Chapter 8, panelists discuss issues surrounding the implementation and use of in-home opioid disposal systems in real-world settings, including opportunities and barriers to disposal, and studies of disposal behaviors. The proceedings concludes in Chapter 9 with panelist and participant reflections on recurring themes from across the workshop. Appendix A contains the workshop agenda and Appendix B contains the biographical sketches of the workshop planning committee members, speakers, and panelists.

---

[2] Comments were accepted through August 28, 2023. See https://www.federalregister.gov/documents/2023/04/04/2023-06650/in-home-disposal-systems-for-opioid-analgesics-request-for-information (accessed November 18, 2023).

2

Life Cycle of Prescribed Opioids

> **Highlights of Key Points Made by Robert Hoffman**
> - Patients are frequently prescribed more doses of an opioid than needed to manage acute or postoperative pain.
> - Patients tend to keep unused opioid medication in the home, and most are not securely stored.
> - Unused prescription opioids have perceived value associated with the costs of obtaining them and the patient's perception of potential future need.
> - Access to opioid analgesics can facilitate non-medical use, diversion, and misuse with potentially fatal outcomes, especially for children who ingest adult doses.
> - Disposal options are available, but people must be willing to give up a product they perceive as useful and for which they have paid.
>
> Presented by Robert Hoffman, June 26, 2023.

Ideally, patients would be prescribed the exact amount of opioid medication needed for management of their pain, they would use all the pills, and they would discard the empty bottle, said Robert Hoffman, professor in the Department of Emergency Medicine at the New York University Grossman School of Medicine. In reality, he says, "patients are frequently prescribed more doses than needed." The unused portion of a prescription has perceived value for many patients, even if it is no longer needed, because of the cost spent to obtain it (including money and time spent to obtain the product itself and the visit to the prescribing provider). Patients tend to keep unused opioid medication in the home, not unlike one might freeze uncooked hamburgers from a barbecue for later use, he suggested. Although harm reduction medicine storage options are available, such as locking pouches or storage cabinets, most unused opioids are simply kept in the bathroom medicine cabinet where they are accessible to anyone who lives in or enters the home.

NON-MEDICAL USE

Easy access to unused opioid medication is a facilitator of non-medical use. Hoffman defined non-medical use as "any use of a prescription product by any individual for the non-intended purpose." This includes use of the prescription product in a different manner, for a different reason, during a different time period, or by a different person than originally prescribed. Examples of non-medical use include using one's own prescribed pain medications to treat pain unrelated to the original prescription, as well as taking another person's unused prescription pain medication for pain relief. He emphasized that non-medical use is potentially fatal. Children are at very high risk of death when exposed to adult doses of opioids, and disparities in child death rates persist, with Hispanic and Black children at increased risk (West et al., 2021).

DIVERSION AND MISUSE

Diversion is when prescription opioids enter the illegal drug market. Diversion can happen anywhere along the product supply chain, including when the patient or someone else with access sells unused prescription opioids to someone else. Hoffman noted that harm reduction approaches such as locked medication pouches or cabinets can be a deterrent to diversion, although it could be the one diverting the product. These harm reduction measures can also be overcome by someone who really desires access.

Hoffman described misuse of opioids as beyond non-medical use, resulting in a cycle of use that can lead to opioid use disorder. "The vast majority of people who misuse prescription drugs get them from someone they know … whether or not there is money involved," Hoffman said (Figure 2-1). The 2019 National Survey on Drug Use and Health reported that 1.6 million people misused a prescription opioid medication for the

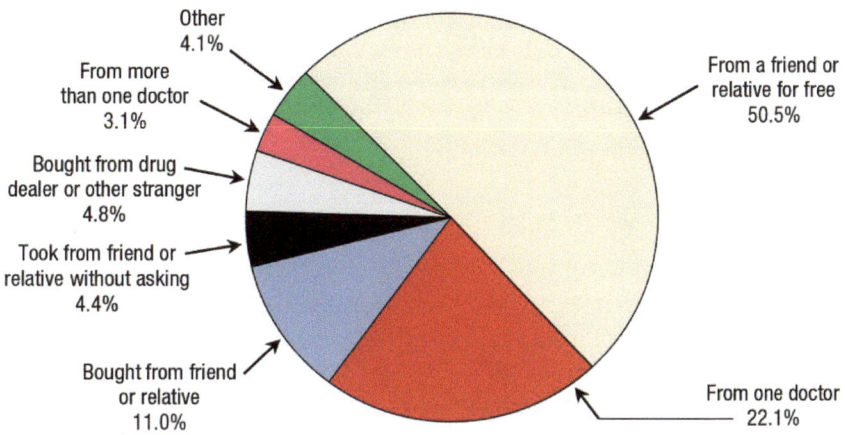

FIGURE 2-1 How misused prescription pain relievers are obtained.
SOURCES: Presented by Robert Hoffman, June 26, 2023; Lipari and Hughes, 2017.

first time that year.[1] Hoffman pointed out that "had it not been available to them, it couldn't have possibly been misused." State-level data on opioid dispensing rates for 2019 suggest that dispensing is highest in six states in the Southeastern United States: West Virginia, Tennessee, Alabama, Missouri, Louisiana, and Arkansas. County-level data, however, clearly show that high levels of dispensing are occurring in pockets of every state, affecting communities nationwide.

DRUG DISPOSAL

Hoffman presented a graphic from FDA with information for the public on three options for disposing of unneeded medication.[2] FDA wants the drugs to be brought to a drug take-back location if available (e.g., on national prescription take-back days, in permanently installed drop boxes). Otherwise, drugs should be flushed if they are on the "FDA flush list" or disposed of in the trash after following instructions for making them unpalatable.

For all disposal options, people must be willing to give up a potentially useful product they have paid for, he reiterated. Although these options seem simple, Hoffman said people often do not understand the directions (e.g., people will put full, closed pill bottles in coffee grounds,

---

[1] See https://www.samhsa.gov/data/report/2019-nsduh-annual-national-report (accessed November 18, 2023).

[2] See https://www.fda.gov/media/111887/download (accessed November 18, 2023).

rather than loose pills). Furthermore, drugs that are flushed or sent to the landfill can contaminate drinking water; opioids have been detected in drinking water samples from across the United States (Skaggs and Logue, 2022). A variety of in-home disposal options are also available, ranging widely in price and ease of use.

INTERVENTION POINTS

Hoffman discussed three points in the life cycle of a prescribed opioid where intervention could prevent adverse outcomes. "Putting the drug out there is the biggest problem," Hoffman said. Appropriate prescribing for pain management can be challenging (which product, how much, for how long). Clinicians must balance reducing unnecessary use with giving patients the pain relief they need. Better non-opioid pain management approaches are needed, he said.

Another point for intervention is home storage of opioids, especially for patients who maintain a supply of opioid medication to manage recurrent or chronic pain, Hoffman said. Risk prevention interventions include secure home storage options and having naloxone available to treat exposures.

The intervention point germane to this workshop is disposal of unused product. Hoffman suggested that in-home disposal systems as an intervention are most likely to be taken up by people who are or can be informed about the risk and/or who are socially conscious. In his practice he has found that it is easier to make the argument for opioid disposal when there are children or teens in the home. It is potentially more difficult to convince patients who face barriers to acquiring the drug to dispose of unused product. Examples of such barriers include cost, health insurance coverage, and geographic location/rurality.

Hoffman reiterated that a significant challenge for uptake and use of in-home disposal systems is convincing people to discard something they paid for, even if they no longer need it. People want self-determination and "expect that they'll have pain in some future moment," he said. He suggested that part of the solution is making health care affordable and accessible to everyone, which he acknowledged is far beyond the scope of this workshop.

There is unlikely to be a one-size-fits-all model for safe opioid disposal, and Hoffman offered several considerations for the development of in-home opioid disposal systems. First, what would motivate people to dispose of something they might consider to be of value, and what type of disposal systems would be acceptable and affordable for users? For the systems themselves, is the device efficient and effective in removing the drug from the community, is it cost effective, and what is the final disposition of the drug in the environment?

3

Envisioning Disposal Systems to Remove Opioids from the Home

> **Highlights of Key Points Made by Individual Speakers***
>
> - In-home opioid disposal systems should be easy to use and provided in a timely manner. (Agarwal, Huang)
> - A number of variables can impact how people make decisions when they interact with packaged products. A human–packaging interaction model could help identify which variables are meaningful when it comes to the design and use of in-home opioid drug disposal systems. (Bix)
> - Timely reminders of the need to dispose of unused opioids are needed, and approaches such as text-based reminders for patients are being studied. (Agarwal, Egan)
> - There is a lack of public awareness about the risk of keeping unused opioids in the home and how to properly dispose of these drug products. (Agarwal, Egan)
> - Those who may be aware of the need to dispose of unused opioids may be thwarted by a lack of useful or accurate information about available disposal options, and confusion about which option to choose. (Baran, Egan)
> - Barriers to the use of opioid disposal systems can include complexity of use, cost, and a desire to hold on to unused drug. (Agarwal, Baran, Egan)

- Implementation of opioid disposal systems is impacted by culture at the patient, provider, health system, and community levels. (Huang)

*This list is the rapporteurs' summary of points made by the individual speakers identified, and the statements have not been endorsed or verified by the National Academies of Sciences, Engineering, and Medicine. They are not intended to reflect a consensus among workshop participants.

DESIGN AND ITS RELATION TO HUMAN BEHAVIOR

Laura Bix, assistant dean for teaching, learning, and academic analytics at Michigan State University College of Agriculture & Natural Resources at Michigan State University, has worked to adapt and combine design models from different fields to manage the multifactorial issues that are involved with human–product interactions. Although her research and regulatory attention are largely focused on how human–package interactions impact behaviors such as medication selection, adherence, or compliance, she said the model could likely be applied to the interactions between humans and drug disposal systems.

Research is available on the extent to which a package may help ensure the safety and efficacy of a given product throughout its defined shelf life. Less attention has been given to the human component, specifically how people interact with a package and how this may impact their decisions and behaviors. Early studies on user-centered design were more qualitative, such as research on user comprehension of labeling. Bix established the Packaging HUB (Healthcare, Universal Design, and Biomechanics) at Michigan State to focus on quantifying the interactions between people and packaging and applying that knowledge to inform policy and package design, with the goal of improving health outcomes.

Five Stages of Information Processing

"For information to be effective, the user must go through five different stages of processing," Bix explained (de la Fuente and Bix, 2011):

- **Exposure** to the information.
- **Perception** of the information through one of the five senses. She noted that interactions with a package or product primarily involve vision.

- **Encodation** of the perceived information by the brain into an electrical signal it can interpret.
- **Comprehension** of the encoded information (e.g., if the information encoded is that the product contains legumes, does a user who has a peanut allergy understand that the product could contain peanuts?).
- **Execution** of a suitable action or behavior based on comprehension of the information.

Bix then noted that the ability to process information provided on a packaged product through the five stages depends on the

- **person** (processing is impacted by experiences, cognitive and physical abilities, beliefs, habits, etc.);
- **context** (environment where the interaction with the information occurs, including distractions and competing tasks);
- **task** (which in the case of a drug could be proper opening, administration, storage, and/or disposal of the packaged drug product); and
- **design of the packaged product.**

Quantifying Consumer Interactions with Product Packaging

Studies by Bix and colleagues offer methods and lessons potentially applicable to the study of patient interaction with opioid disposal systems. One study discussed by Bix evaluated the extent to which over-the-counter (OTC) drug labeling about tamper-evident features and the lack of child-resistant packaging was prominent and conspicuous, as required by law (Bix et al., 2009). The eye movements of study participants were observed as they considered five different OTCs for purchase to determine how they interacted with five key pieces of information: "brand name, indications, drug facts label, child-resistant warning which indicates not for households with young children, and the warning alerting to tamper-evident features," she said. One finding she highlighted was that, across all five OTC packages, more than 80 percent of participants did not look at the warning regarding tamper-evident features. She pointed out that any efforts to ensure the tamper-evident messaging on the product label was understandable were irrelevant because most people were not looking at that warning.

In another study, participants considered whether mock brands of OTC drugs were appropriate for them based on how the (fake) brand name, active ingredient, and indications were displayed on the package (Liu, 2016). Of 82 participants, 8 percent looked at the drug facts label for every product package when deciding if they would purchase the product or not, while 62 percent never looked at the drug facts label on any of the packages.

A study of tamper-evident solutions for a food puree found that consumers could not be relied on to notice tampering or to act appropriately when they did notice tampering. The "consumers" were experts in biosystems engineering and packaging at Michigan State. When presented with the packaged puree that had been tampered with, the expert consumers were less likely to find the tampering if it was not near the container closure. Furthermore, all the experts reported having used products in their personal lives that had "a failed induction seal or a failed shrink sleeve over a product," Bix said. Some reported not wanting to make another trip to the store to try to exchange; others reasoned that "machinery is inconsistent," "seals pop off," or "things happen in transit." The proposal stemming from this study was to design a barcode with color-changing ink that could respond to "changes in the headspace gas" and make the barcode unreadable. This approach would prevent the consumer from buying the tampered product. Bix suggested that a similar approach might be considered for opioids, perhaps some process that might "slowly render the product inert."

User-Centered Design

Numerous independent variables can potentially impact how people make decisions when they interact with packaged products. The model discussed can help to identify and assess which variables are most meaningful to study and target for intervention. Bix emphasized the importance of understanding where a system design is failing, and developing new solutions that address root causes (e.g., is it a perception problem, a comprehension problem, an execution problem?).

"Even when you create a design that is successful through processing, consumers/patients may behave in ways incongruent to what you desire/intend," Bix concluded, and she suggested considering designs that do not depend on consumer behavior.

DESIGNING USABLE IN-HOME OPIOID DISPOSAL SYSTEMS

The International Organization for Standardization definition of usability considers the effectiveness, efficiency, and satisfaction a system affords the user, Bix said. Following the presentation, Bix was joined by four panelists for a discussion of characteristics of usable in-home opioid disposal systems, barriers to their implementation and use, and health equity considerations in the development of in-home disposal systems. Panelists included Anish Agarwal, assistant professor of emergency medicine at the University of Pennsylvania Perelman School of Medicine; Lindsay Baran, senior research director in the Health Care Evaluation department at NORC at the University of Chicago; Kathleen Egan, assistant professor in the Department of Health Education and Promotion at East Carolina University; and Lyen Huang, assistant professor of surgery at the University of Utah Spencer Fox Eccles School of Medicine. The discussion was moderated by Ruchi Fitzgerald, assistant professor at Rush University and service chief of inpatient addiction medicine at PCC Community Wellness Center.

Characteristics of Usable In-Home Opioid Disposal Systems

From his perspective as an emergency medicine clinician and health care innovator, Agarwal said in-home opioid disposal systems need to be easy to use and provided in a time-sensitive manner. Agarwal described a study in which patients are engaged via text messaging during the week following their surgery (Agarwal et al., 2021). Participants report their use of the prescribed opioid and their pain score and are reminded "in rapid, real-time fashion" when it is appropriate to dispose of unused drug. Agarwal then described a follow-up randomized controlled trial (RCT) in which, in addition to the text messaging, in-home disposal systems were mailed to participants to arrive when it was predicted they would no longer be taking the prescribed opioids (most frequently timed to arrive 4 to 5 days postoperatively) (Agarwal et al., 2022). Feedback from patients indicated that they receive a large packet of information upon discharge and often forget about any information on the need to dispose of unused opioids at some future time. The study found that patients who were postoperatively mailed easy-to-use disposal kits and received text message reminders to dispose were "twice as likely to dispose," he said.

Egan agreed with the need for more timely disposal messaging and said she is also studying a text message intervention that reminds patients to dispose as they near the end of their prescription (Egan et al., 2020). A challenge, she noted, is the wide variability in prescription length. Huang also emphasized the importance of the timing of interventions. University of Utah Health provides free disposal kits to all patients who fill a benzodiazepine or opioid prescription. Huang's studies of real-world use of in-home opioid disposal kits have found that there is intent to dispose but not follow-through (Huang et al., 2023). Postoperative follow-up surveys indicated that 51 percent of patients want to or plan to dispose, but at 2 weeks postsurgery only 26 percent have actually done so. Huang highlighted the need to address patient-level barriers to disposal and to better target messaging.

Barriers to Safe Disposal of Unused Opioids

Egan shared lessons from her experience working with community coalitions to address substance use and expand disposal opportunities. She said recurrent feedback from community members is that there is a lack of awareness and education about the need to dispose of opioids and how they should be disposed (including the use of disposal systems). Agarwal also emphasized the need to communicate the risk that opioids present for others in the patient's home and in the community, and the importance of disposing of unused drug.

People who recognize the risk of having opioids in the home "are more likely to be interested in disposal and actually dispose," Egan said. There are concerns, however, about the safety of the disposal systems themselves, and the potential danger to children or animals that encounter or ingest the systems. In addition, those who are aware of the need to dispose are often "immobilized by all the options." For those who decide to go to a take-back location, for example, the DEA list of public disposal boxes is often inaccurate. She explained that pharmacies must register to have a disposal box, but they might not install a box or might remove an existing box. Community feedback suggests that people will try to dispose at a pharmacy one time. If there is no disposal box or the box is closed, they are unmotivated to try again, she said. Baran agreed with Egan that lack of awareness is a main barrier, and that many people not only are unaware of existing drug disposal options but also struggle to find accurate information. An Internet search for "how to get rid of unneeded opioids" nets wide-ranging results. There is valuable information from reputable sources such as federal websites about disposal options, Baran said, "but for the average person who is just looking for a clear answer about how to get rid of their medication, it's incredibly complicated to navigate."

Barriers to using some of the opioid disposal options that are available include complexity of the disposal system, costs, and in some cases, the need to travel to a disposal location, which Baran noted requires transportation and has costs. Egan said there is feedback from communities that the cost of opioid disposal systems is a significant barrier to uptake. While there might be interest in having a disposal kit, people are generally not willing to pay for it, she said. Egan also noted that kits might not be used to dispose of opioids. She described one intervention in which community members were provided with a packaged disposal system (in this case, the Deterra system). Most found the disposal system easy to use, but further analysis revealed that many intended to use the system to dispose of drugs other than opioids.

Another barrier to disposal of unused opioids is that, for a variety of reasons, some people do not want to dispose of them, Baran said. She reiterated the point by Robert Hoffman that people are often unwilling to give up something they paid for, even if they no longer need it, because they believe they might need it in the future. In this regard, barriers to accessing prescription opioid medications for pain management are a barrier to disposal. Agarwal said that when informed about the need for disposal, his patients often raise concerns about possibly needing their pain medication in the future. Baran said people, especially those with episodic pain conditions, often have "a justified fear" of not being able to obtain additional medication if needed.

Huang said that when envisioning in-home disposal of opioids, it is important to acknowledge the culture at the patient, provider, health system, and community levels in which implementation is being attempted. For example, he said that algorithms and electronic health record (EHR) prompts designed to help clinicians reduce opioid prescribing have been implemented, "but the most challenging part has been convincing attending surgeons to go along with this low- or no-opioid prescribing." Medical residents have reported wanting to avoid prescribing opioids at discharge when the patient has not taken any for 48 hours, but they often prescribe anyway out of concern that the patient will call later with pain or the attending will be displeased that nothing was prescribed. Convincing patients they do not need opioids "just in case" is another cultural barrier to both prescribing and disposal.

In addressing barriers, Bix said it is important to identify which behaviors need to be motivated and in what situations, understanding that "people are incredibly unpredictable." She reiterated the importance of empirical evaluation of the system to identify where it is failing and to address the root causes. Huang said research is needed on which types of interventions can successfully motivate the desired opioid disposal behaviors.

Targeting In-Home Disposal Interventions

Panelists discussed whether to focus on particular subgroups for in-home disposal interventions. Egan said that patients treating chronic pain tend to use up their medication within the prescribed period, and harm reduction strategies discussed by Hoffman, such as secure storage, are needed. Baran proposed thinking about subgroups based on prescribing practice (e.g., short term versus long term) rather than on condition (e.g., chronic versus acute). Chronic and acute pain are not distinct subgroups and there are overlaps. As an example, she shared that she personally has a chronic pain condition but does not use opioids on a chronic basis. An opioid might be prescribed short term, for example, if she were to have surgery to address an acute flare of her condition. Baran also suggested that in-home disposal is a "universal prevention intervention," but outcomes and measures of success might be population specific. For example, a reduction in child poisonings might be one measure of success of the uptake of in-home disposal of opioids by parents.

Agarwal highlighted the need to understand the "blind spots" in prescribing. He observed that patients are often prescribed a particular dose and duration of opioid for an injury or after surgery because that is the dose and duration that has always been used. It is not possible to know who will need more pain management after a procedure and who might need none. But prescribers want to know when their patients are in pain, Agarwal said, and his group is studying a real-time communication mechanism to report pain management concerns from patients to their surgeons and other prescribers. This type of communication is a change in the culture of prescribing, he said. Furthermore, "surgeons are profoundly trusted resources for patients," and can inform patients about the risks of opioids in the home and encourage them to dispose of unused medication using a provided in-home disposal kit. He discussed developing a learning health system to inform prescribing guidelines that better anticipate patient pain management needs and tailor prescribing accordingly, and provide timely information, reminders, and supplies for disposal.

Rather than focusing on particular subgroups for disposal interventions, Huang suggested taking a patient-centered approach to disposal. The capability exists to collect feedback from individual patients about real and perceived barriers to their disposal of their unused opioids and provide "very targeted interventions that address those concerns," he said. In essence, this is "disposal intervention as personalized medicine," he added.

Health Equity Considerations

R. Fitzgerald raised the issue of health equity in the development and implementation of in-home opioid disposal systems. Key considerations for equitable access to disposal systems include the cost and ease of acquiring the disposal system, Baran said. For example, is the disposal kit provided when the medication is dispensed, or does the patient have to travel again or elsewhere to acquire it or pay to have it shipped? Are additional supplies required? Raising awareness of the need to dispose of unused opioids and of the options available is also a component of ensuring equitable access. As discussed, ease of use is an important feature of any disposal system for use by the public, but this feature might be especially important for individuals who are homeless or not in a traditional home setting. The systems, including the instructions, should be both cognitively and physically accessible, Baran continued. For example, instructions should be clear, and the process should not require many steps or take much dexterity or manual effort (e.g., mixing). She suggested that having support available from a pharmacist, prescribing physician, or perhaps a toll-free number would also be helpful. In summary, Baran said systems should be "easy to access; free or low-cost … easy to explain and easy to use with little room for error;" and safe for users, children, pets, and the environment. Egan shared feedback from the communities she works with that many find the instructions for disposing of opioids challenging to follow. She added that accessibility includes making the font large enough for older users to see.

Bix suggested that the efficiency component of usability is a key measure for designing equitable and accessible in-home opioid disposal systems. Efficiency addresses whether the user has the resources needed to realize the outcome the product is intended to facilitate, she said. These resources could be physical strength, cognition, ability to follow the steps required, ability to travel, and access to transportation, for example. Different populations might face different usability challenges. In designing a product, it is important to understand at the outset which population the product is intended for and what behavior it is intended to motivate, Bix said.

Egan reported that implementation of disposal kiosks at pharmacies throughout communities in North Carolina was equitable to the extent that it did not vary by the zip code of the pharmacies. Variability in implementation of disposal kiosks was associated with the type of pharmacy, due to factors that Egan said could also translate to variability in the dispensing of in-home disposal kits. Pharmacists in corporate-owned pharmacies said cost is not a factor in the implementation disposal kiosks, but the managing pharmacist does not have control over whether a kiosk is installed in their pharmacy. Independent pharmacists reported that cost is a barrier, and installation of a disposal kiosk is often supported by external funding. Huang agreed there can be challenges of providing resources to patients through pharmacies and said pathways are needed to ensure that distribution is not limited to large-chain pharmacies or large health systems for whom cost is not a barrier. Egan added that community substance use coalitions are using funding from the ONDCP Drug Free Communities program to distribute in-home disposal kits, but there are not yet outcomes data to assess whether this approach is making an impact.

Agarwal pointed out that unequal access to digital technology and digital health could impact equitable implementation of disposal kits. He suggested looking for opportunities to place disposal resources in accessible places (as has been done with the placement of Narcan in libraries in Philadelphia and needle drop boxes in airport restrooms).

Huang said rurality impacts access to health care providers, pharmacies, and disposal kiosks. He pointed out that "rural" is subjective. In the mountain west where he lives, patients often travel 5 or 6 hours for health care or more than an hour to the nearest pharmacy, which can be "over a mountain range that's inaccessible in the middle of wintertime because of the wind and snow." Huang said the timed mailing of disposal kits, as done in the study by Agarwal, could be a challenge in rural areas for patients who do not have a traditional mailing address (as is the case on some Tribal reservations). Rurality also impacts pain management, he said. While a provider can promise to remotely prescribe a new or refill prescription when the patient needs it, the patient might not be able to go to the pharmacy to pick it up.

Lessons from Naloxone Distribution

Agarwal drew a parallel between distribution of naloxone and distribution of in-home disposal systems in that the goal of both is to provide something to the patient that will not be used right away. He conducted a study which found that most patients who were dispensed naloxone spray at discharge from the emergency department were carrying it with them in the week after discharge. By contrast, most patients who were discharged with a prescription for naloxone were not carrying it, and the need to go and fill the prescription seemed to be a barrier. Egan shared feedback from a pharmacist who reported that even a small copay of $4 dissuaded people from filling a prescription for naloxone. She suggested that patients would also be unlikely to accept a copay for an in-home disposal kit. Huang described efforts to increase distribution of naloxone across Utah. A challenge has been that patients "overwhelmingly prefer the nasal spray version versus injection form," he said, but the spray can cost patients hundreds of dollars out of pocket, and many do not pick it up from the pharmacy. R. Fitzgerald noted that the availability of naloxone varies by state and locality and is available to everyone free of cost in Illinois.

4

The Role of In-Home Opioid Disposal

Highlights of Key Points Made by Individual Speakers*

- There is no one-size-fits-all solution when it comes to reducing the risk of opioid misuse in the home. A multifaceted approach is needed that incorporates education, a range of disposal options, and safe storage options. (Compton, Egan, Gaw, Horwitz)
- Achieving a shift in cultural and social norms around opioid storage and disposal behaviors will require repeated, targeted, easy-to-understand education provided by trusted sources along the health care pathway and community partners. (Gaw, Horwitz, Sherman)
- Unified, context-appropriate messaging is needed about the risks of having opioids in the home and the role of in-home disposal in reducing those risks. (Horwitz, Morones, Sherman)
- Key partners, including consumers, should be engaged in developing the messaging intended to promote disposal behaviors. (Egan)
- Some areas where empirical research is needed include understanding patient decision making; exploring motivating disposal behaviors; studying effective communication strategies; conducting comparative effectiveness studies, including

usefulness in reducing diversion; and developing methods for implementation. (Compton)
- It is important to recognize that when people use an in-home opioid disposal system, they may dispose of other types of drugs in addition to opioids. (Egan)

*This list is the rapporteurs' summary of points made by the individual speakers identified, and the statements have not been endorsed or verified by the National Academies of Sciences, Engineering, and Medicine. They are not intended to reflect a consensus among workshop participants.

FACILITATING IN-HOME DISPOSAL OF OPIOID ANALGESICS

Following on her comments during the panel session, Kathleen Egan discussed her research on facilitating in-home disposal of opioid analgesics in greater detail.

Community Member Beliefs About Disposal

Egan summarized her findings from two studies of community member perceptions about opioid disposal, which were done to inform the development of interventions to facilitate disposal (Helme et al., 2020; Otufowora et al., 2023[1]). Together, these studies encompassed 22 focus groups that included a total of 130 patients who had been prescribed opioids. Egan listed shared findings across the studies, including the following:

- **"Lack of awareness and education about disposal options."** Egan noted that the first study focused on perceptions about disposal boxes, which she said were generally only available at law enforcement agencies at that time (Helme et al., 2020). The second study assessed awareness and perceptions of the range of disposal options on the FDA website, including in-home disposal systems (Otufowora et al., 2023). When people do dispose, they will use both in-home options and take-back sites. Egan further pointed out that disposal programs vary by region, and that neither study asked whether patients used mail-back envelopes because it is not generally an option in North Carolina, where she conducted the study.

---

[1] Preparation of a manuscript describing this study was in progress at the time of the workshop. It has since been accepted for publication.

- **"Confusion about 'best' disposal option immobilizes patients."** Egan said study participants often reported keeping opioids in the home because they did not feel there was a suitable option for disposal (e.g., some did not feel flushing was acceptable).
- **"Desire to choose the disposal option that is best for them," despite reported confusion.** Factors participants reported taking into consideration included "convenience and accessibility, cost, distrust in law enforcement agencies, [and] environmental concerns."
- **Perception that disposing of unused opioids protects household members.** Egan noted that some participants who were more motivated to dispose had children, pets, or a person at risk for substance misuse in the home.
- **Desire to retain unused opioid analgesics "just in case."**

Studying Interventions to Facilitate Disposal

Distribution of In-Home Disposal Systems

Egan elaborated on a pilot study focused on distribution (Otufowora et al., 2023). Community health workers distributed in-home disposal systems through a local community outreach program and provided education about use. Of the 124 individuals who reported use of opioid medication, 100 percent accepted the offered in-home disposal system, and 98 percent of those said they "expected use to be very easy or somewhat easy." However, "only about 50 percent intended to use it to dispose of opioid medication," Egan said.

Raising Awareness of Disposal Boxes

Another study assessed public response to proposed interventions intended to increase awareness of the need to dispose of opioids promptly in drop boxes (Egan et al., 2020). To inform a communications campaign by local health departments, campaign materials were pretested in focus groups using a "forced exposure, cross-sectional survey design," Egan said. The development of eight messages with visuals was informed by the health beliefs identified in the study by Helme and colleagues (2020). Egan emphasized the importance of including key partners and said experts in health communication were engaged in developing the materials to be tested.

Egan shared study findings for three of the visual messages, which illustrate the importance of engaging patients as partners as well. Showing study participants messaging centered on a photo of a small child with medications loose on a table in front of them "elicited the strongest perceptions and beliefs that disposal would be beneficial to their household," Egan reported. Messaging with an image of someone using a local disposal box scored well in promoting beliefs of self-efficacy (i.e., participants had confidence they knew how to dispose) but did not motivate interest in disposing. Messaging with a photo of an adolescent taking pills from a medicine cabinet was not perceived as intended (i.e., as diversion), and participants believed the person in the photo could be an adult or could be about to take their own prescribed medication. The campaign has now been implemented, but data on any impact are not available.

Text-Based Prompts to Encourage Secure Storage and Disposal of Opioids

Egan is currently designing an RCT to assess the efficacy and feasibility of using text messaging to prompt opioid storage and disposal behaviors after patients have filled a prescription. The RCT will leverage the automated text messaging systems used by pharmacies to send messages about secure storage, followed by messages that prompt disposal of unused opioids at some yet-to-be defined point.

The development of the study intervention is participant-driven, Egan said, with the text messages informed by focus groups and pretested using a cross-sectional forced exposure design. Focus groups considered proposed text messages relating to disposal through iterative rounds of review, responding to questions about their understanding of a message, how it impacted their perceptions, and whether it would motivate them to dispose. Egan pointed out that the five final messages chosen for pretesting based on user input were not the messages the research team used at the start. She emphasized that developing messaging for the public without consumer feedback can result in a campaign with "messages that don't end up resonating with our end user."

Three text messages pertaining to disposal were selected from the pretesting to be included in the RCT. Based on focus group input, Egan said that text-based disposal prompts will also include an embedded image with information about how to dispose. "Participants said they don't want to click on a link to a website to go find this information," she reported. She added that, in the absence of a standard of care, the control group in the RCT will receive a delayed intervention.

From Policy to Implementation:
Lessons from Pharmacy-Based Disposal Boxes

A study by Egan found that the number of pharmacies with drug disposal boxes in North Carolina increased from 1.7 percent in 2016 to 13.5 percent in 2021 (Egan et al., 2022). She said, however, that

"13.5 percent is not enough for the populations that need these disposal boxes." She reported that uptake of disposal boxes in 2016 was predominantly by independently owned pharmacies, done in partnership with substance use prevention coalitions. Today, the pharmacies most likely to have disposal boxes are corporate chain pharmacies. Egan observed that deimplementation of disposal boxes is occurring in all types of pharmacies. In the case of independently owned pharmacies, the boxes tend to be deimplemented when external funding support for them runs out.

Egan shared findings from interviews with pharmacists about disposal boxes, which she said could translate to in-home disposal systems should pharmacists be responsible for dispensing. Pharmacists believed that "disposal options meet patients' needs" and that "their patients benefit from these programs," she reported. Some pharmacists believed disposal efforts were "part of their scope of work" and that they benefited from these programs as well. Pharmacists in corporate-owned pharmacies said there is no cost or operational burden to them, while independent pharmacists and small chains face cost burdens that can make continued implementation unsustainable. When looking to partner with pharmacies to implement disposal boxes, it is important to recognize that pharmacists in corporate pharmacies are unable to make any changes to their pharmacy. Independently owned and operated pharmacies expressed interest in working with community partners to implement disposal boxes, Egan said, but showed concern about expiration of funding. From an implementation perspective, Egan summarized, it is important to consider what assistance those who will be implementing disposal policies might need to successfully provide disposal options, such as funding or educational materials. If disposal systems are dispensed in the context of care, she noted the need to consider whether dispensing might need to have a protocol or whether an ICD (*International Classification of Diseases*)-10 code would be needed.

In closing, Egan said there is no one-size-fits-all solution to reducing the risk of opioids in the home. A comprehensive approach is needed that incorporates education, disposal systems for patients who have unused opioids, and secure storage options for patients who need to retain opioids.

CONSIDERING THE ROLES OF IN-HOME DISPOSAL

Following the presentation, Egan was joined by four panelists for further discussion of the role of an ideal in-home opioid disposal system in mitigating the risk of prescription opioid misuse or overdose. Panelists included Christopher Gaw, a pediatric emergency medicine fellow and associate fellow at the Center for Injury Research and Prevention at the Children's Hospital of Philadelphia; Jeff Horwitz, chief executive officer of the Stop the Addiction Fatality Epidemic (SAFE) Project; Susan Sherman, Bloomberg Professor of American Health in the Department of Health, Behavior and Society at Johns Hopkins Bloomberg School of Public Health; and Wilson Compton, deputy director of the National Institute on Drug Abuse (NIDA) at the National Institutes of Health. The discussion was moderated by Robert Morones, area injury prevention specialist at Indian Health Service (IHS) Phoenix Area.

Preventing Pediatric Injury and Death

The Poison Prevention Packaging Act in 1970 required systematic changes to medication packaging, which led to "a 40 to 50 percent reduction in injury exposures and fatalities in the pediatric population," Gaw said. However, data from CDC, the National Poison Data System, and child death reviews show that an increasing number of pediatric injuries and fatalities are associated with opioids (Gaw et al., 2023). In young children, exposure to opioids is generally associated with exploratory behavior, while exposure in teens is frequently experimental. Most pediatric injury from opioid exposure is accidental, although Gaw added that some cases of pediatric opioid injury are intentional or associated with child abuse.

Gaw said in-home drug disposal systems could play a role in pediatric injury prevention efforts. "If you have no exposure to an opioid, you should theoretically have no injury or fatality from an opioid," he said. However, to be effective they must be used. Furthermore, the risk persists until the drug is disposed of, which cannot be done until use as prescribed is completed. He highlighted the need for "a multifaceted and a multipronged approach" that includes education and safe storage options. Effecting a shift in cultural and social norms around storage and disposal behaviors will require repeated, targeted, easy-to-understand messaging provided by different sources, Gaw said. As an example, he said the use of seatbelts and child car seats is now a social norm and essentially automatic behavior, but it took decades of public health messaging. Morones likened a parent/guardian protecting children by securing them in a motor vehicle to protecting them by securing and disposing of drugs in the home.

As discussed by Egan, there can be challenges in moving from policy to implementation. Gaw said that policies around pediatric injury prevention can be ineffective or potentially harmful if stakeholders do not understand them or do not believe they are necessary. Current data on pediatric injury from opioid exposure are primarily raw epidemiologic data. Additional research is needed to better understand the pathways to pediatric exposure and injury, and whether and how parents will use in-home disposal systems.

Preventing Fatal Opioid Overdoses

In 2022, more than 100,000 people in the United States died from overdoses, Horwitz said, or nearly 300 people per day.[2] A recent study found that having an opioid in the home is associated with a 60 percent increased risk of overdose by someone for whom it was not prescribed (Hendricks et al., 2023). Furthermore, Horwitz said that "the majority of 12th graders will say they've experimented … in their own medicine cabinet," and "80 percent of heroin users today will self-admit that they started out with misuse in their home." Many are under the misperception that because a drug is a prescription drug, it is safe for them.

The SAFE Project was created by a family following the fatal overdose of their son and operates under the premise that creating change requires collaboration and collective action.[3] Horwitz said the SAFE Project considers in-home opioid disposal solutions to have a role in expanding the number of options available for patients to remove opioid drugs from their home.

With support from in-kind donations from manufacturers, the SAFE Project has distributed about 140,000 in-home disposal systems over the past 5 years, Horwitz said. Through follow-up surveys, he said that 80 to 90 percent of those who accepted a disposal system reported using it. He added that in cases where a disposal pouch had been offered and declined, providing an explanation of why it is needed and how to use it frequently leads to acceptance.

Harm Reduction

Sherman defined harm reduction as "a set of practical strategies and ideas aimed at reducing the negative consequences associated with drug use." A principle of harm reduction is acknowledging that people misuse drugs. Programs and tools are aimed at reducing the risks of associated harms, such as overdose or becoming infected with HIV or hepatitis C. Examples of harm reduction programs and tools mentioned by Sherman include "syringe service programs, naloxone, [and] drug-checking technologies like fentanyl test strips."

---

[2] See https://www.cdc.gov/nchs/nvss/vsrr/drug-overdose-data.htm (accessed November 11, 2023).
[3] See https://www.safeproject.us/ (accessed November 11, 2023).

Social justice is a tenet of harm reduction, working with people to understand their experience and designing and implementing programs, tools, and messaging centered on that experience. In this regard Sherman pointed out the need to consider the use of "in-home" disposal systems and other disposal options by those who are unhoused. Another principle is "not to otherize and dehumanize people," Sherman said. She added that it is important to reduce the stigma associated with the use of opioids so that people are more willing to accept a disposal system when offered or to bring drugs to a public take-back location.

She suggested that the concept of harm reduction can also provide lessons for in-home drug disposal with regard to reducing harms to the environments where opioid disposal systems are used and discarded (e.g., homes, landfills).

Research Needs

Misuse and diversion of prescription opioids remains a significant problem that has yet to be solved, Compton said, but it is also important to note that use of illicit opioid drugs is rapidly increasing (e.g., counterfeits of prescription medications, heroin, synthetic opioids such as fentanyl). He highlighted several areas where research is needed to understand the role of in-home disposal systems in the larger portfolio of options intended to reduce circulation of unused prescription opioids. NIDA supports some research in this area, such as the study on messaging discussed by Egan (above).

One area where NIDA believes research would be helpful is in understanding decision making by potential users of in-home drug disposal systems. This includes research on how to directly influence uptake of disposal systems as well as indirect effects of providing in-home drug disposal options, he said. For example, he suggested that providing a disposal kit is itself a strong message that there is danger in retaining an opioid. Even if people choose not to use the provided kit, does having been provided the kit influence their decision to dispose by some other method? Compton said the target is changing behavior so that the practice of disposal becomes essentially automatic (i.e., does not require a cognitive decision). Therefore, research is also needed on effective communication strategies and messaging.

"Understanding the costs and effectiveness of in-home drug disposal as part of a broad range of approaches is a very complicated area," Compton said, and implementation research and economic research are also needed. He suggested that studies and modeling of approaches to address the overdose crisis could include in-home drug disposal systems in the research. Comparative effectiveness studies of in-home drug disposal to other approaches are also needed. Compton agreed with Egan that there will not be a one-size-fits-all solution and said, "Having a broad range of approaches provides the best approach to public health."

The extent to which a disposal approach reduces diversion is another question for empirical research to inform public health decisions about implementation of disposal options. Diversion will be a concern regardless of disposal approach, Compton said, and the issue is how much we can minimize it. Some current in-home disposal systems might make opioids inaccessible for use. While it is "theoretically possible to reconstitute substances from at least some approaches to in-home disposal," there is no empirical data on the extent to which that happens. It will take a significant amount of expertise to retrieve or reconstitute the drug after disposal, but Compton said more research is needed here as well. In his experience as an addiction specialist, Compton said he has observed surprising creativity by patients seeking drugs. He suggested monitoring communication modalities used by illicit drug markets, and drug-using communities could provide information about new approaches to undermine the effectiveness of disposal strategies.

From a primary prevention perspective, Egan said, the goal of disposal is to remove unneeded opioids from the home in a timely manner, and disposal systems can do that. Assessing the outcomes of primary prevention is much more difficult and occurs over the longer term. In this case, research is needed to determine the extent to which disposing of unused opioids prevents substance misuse. She added that there is anecdotal evidence on the unintended consequences of using different disposal options (e.g., the impact of flushing), but quantitative data are lacking.

Messaging and Education

Much of the panel discussion expanded on messaging about the role of in-home disposal of opioids. Panelists discussed the need to educate providers and the public about currently available disposal options while continuing to develop and assess a range of new options.

Horwitz said education is needed, not just about how to use the disposal system but to raise awareness and provide a unified message that having opioid medications in the home presents a risk for everyone there (including pets), and people can reduce that risk by removing the medications from the home. Sherman agreed with the need for practitioners to incorporate unified messaging about opioid use and disposal into their practice. She clarified that unified does not mean the same. Messaging can be tailored to the population and context. Morones agreed and said that for Tribal communities, "water is a precious resource" and people are generally unwilling to flush medications. Messaging about disposal needs to take this context into account.

Horwitz also emphasized the need to consider what message is being conveyed when providing education about current disposal options. He suggested that it is somewhat dismissive to tell people opioids are dangerous drugs but that they can just flush them down the toilet, put them out at the street with the trash mixed into some kitty litter, or send them back through the USPS. In response to a question, Horwitz acknowledged that mail-back envelopes can be an option for those without access to other take-back options, such as those living in rural areas or those who choose not to go to a take-back site, but added that in-home disposal could be an option for them as well. He said a range of options should be made available to enable patients to be successful at disposing of unused opioids.

Egan observed that current messaging asks patients to choose a disposal option based on what is available to them. She suggested that messaging might be better framed around having patients choose which disposal approach best reduces the potential risk to their household. That choice might be based on whether there are young children or someone with substance use disorder in the home, for example.

Gaw said although the clinician and pharmacist are logical potential counseling points, there are practical challenges. An adult primary care encounter with the physician can last 15 to 25 minutes, while a pediatric well check can include only 10 to 15 minutes with the pediatrician, he said. Given the many other competing priorities, including addressing patient and parent concerns, this might not be the most effective venue for fitting in general messaging about opioid safety. Gaw said pediatricians do screen children for risks in the home and provide education and resources accordingly (e.g., pediatric screening for access to a gun in the home is now a protocol at the Children's Hospital of Philadelphia). Pediatric practices are becoming increasingly aware of the need to provide counseling and interventions to mitigate the risks of medications in the home. He noted that no single approach is sufficient, and injury prevention works best in layers.

Pharmacists face similar time constraints on patient interactions. Gaw and Compton both observed that a prescription pickup is often reduced to a card swipe, tapping acknowledgment of a paragraph on a screen that few people read, and a signature. Horwitz acknowledged the challenges but emphasized the importance of taking all opportunities to impart the message that unused opioids present a serious risk. Physicians can mention when prescribing an opioid that they are also going to make sure the patient has an in-home disposal system or whatever option is available regionally, and pharmacists can mention again when dispensing that disposal is important. If everyone reinforces the message, "the behavior will follow," he said.

In addition to identifying communication opportunities across the life cycle of prescribed opioids (e.g., the prescriber, someone else in the prescriber's office, the health care system, the dispenser), Compton said broad community-based communication strategies about opioid risks are also needed to prime the public for more successful uptake of messaging from health care providers. Gaw agreed that community partners have a role to play in providing effective messaging about opioids and preparing patients to discuss concerns with a trusted provider. He suggested leveraging social media to engage target audiences and looking to other novel communication approaches. Sherman also agreed with the need to intervene at multiple points across the opioid prescribing pathway and with the need to engage a range of community partners. She suggested engaging harm reduction outreach workers, syringe service programs, or homeless organizations as well. While this might seem counterintuitive, she said that they often work with people who quit using opioids and would need disposal options.

Panelists also discussed the complex association of messaging, perceptions, and behavior. Hanz Atia, a policy and programs associate at the Product Stewardship Institute (PSI), raised the issue of children exploring in-home disposal pouches before the opioids have been fully deactivated, and whether perceptions that the system is non-toxic might lead parents to be less careful with the used pouch. Gaw said that having the opioids in a disposal system, even if not yet fully unavailable for use, is generally still better than the alternative of a child having access to intact drug. Parental perception of the safety of disposal systems is an important factor in willingness to use them. The final product–drug mixture should be non-toxic. A challenge is addressing the potential lack of understanding of the time that might be required for full deactivation and the potential for real or perceived harm. If there is widespread perception that the system or end mixture is harmful, efforts to implement in-home disposal could be hampered. Conversely, the product–drug mixture is intended to be non-toxic, but it is not known if this information might impart a false sense of security prior to full drug deactivation and lead some to be less cautious with the used disposal system.

5

Risk Evaluation and Mitigation Strategy (REMS)

> **Highlights of Key Points Made by Lynn Mehler**
>
> - A risk evaluation and mitigation strategy (REMS) is a tool that can be used to mitigate serious safety risks of a product to the extent necessary for the product to be approvable.
> - The Food and Drug Administration (FDA) has the authority to require a REMS as part of product approval as well as at any time after approval, and to require the inclusion of specific elements to assure safe use.
> - FDA's expanded REMS authority under the SUPPORT Act allows the agency to require interventions (e.g., packaging, disposal systems) to mitigate a serious risk.
> - The product sponsor is responsible for ensuring the compliance of prescribers, dispensers, and patients with the REMS.
>
> Presented by Lynn Mehler, June 27, 2023.

Lynn Mehler, partner at Hogan Lovells LLP, practice area lead for pharmaceuticals and biotechnology, provided a legal and practical overview of REMS.

FDA can require a REMS "if it determines that it is necessary to mitigate a specific risk to ensure the product benefits outweigh its risk," Mehler said. In essence, a REMS is a tool that can be used to mitigate seri-

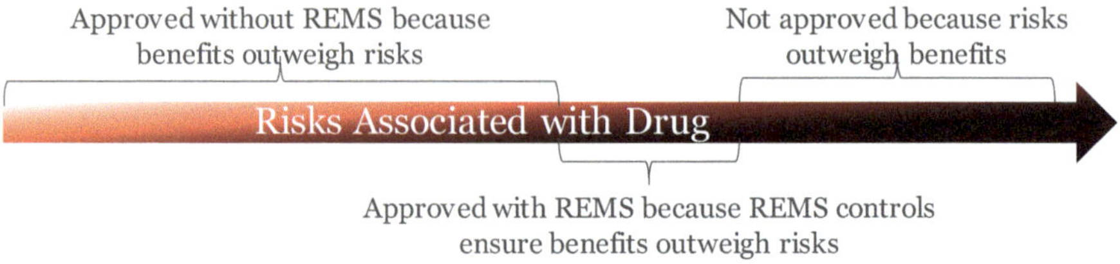

FIGURE 5-1 Risk-based drug approval continuum.
NOTE: REMS = risk evaluation and mitigation strategy.
SOURCE: Presented by Lynn Mehler, June 27, 2023.

ous safety risks of a product to the extent necessary for the product to be approvable (Figure 5-1).

In considering whether to require or modify a REMS, FDA is required by statute to "consider whether the REMS unduly burdens patient access and attempt to minimize the burden on the health care delivery system," Mehler said. FDA has the authority to require a REMS as part of product approval as well as at any time after approval, and to require the inclusion of specific elements to assure safe use (ETASU). ETASU can include requirements for certification of prescribers and pharmacists, conditions for dispensing "only in certain health care settings" or "only with documentation of safe-use conditions," and requirements for patient monitoring and enrollment in a registry.

All REMS must be assessed periodically to ensure they continue to meet the stated goals and consider whether modifications are needed. Mehler described this as an "iterative [and] complicated process." If the sponsor is found to be out of compliance with the REMS requirements, the drug is considered to be misbranded, and FDA will take enforcement action, which can include "civil monetary penalties, withdrawal of approval, or criminal liabilities."[1] Per the statute, the sponsor is responsible for ensuring the compliance of prescribers, dispensers, and patients with the REMS. Mehler said there is a process for handling noncompliance by stakeholders (with decertification of prescribers or dispensers only as a "last resort").

---

[1] Mehler explained that "a drug is misbranded if its label or labeling are false or misleading in any way (including REMS materials)."

REMS FORMAT AND CONTENT

A REMS has two main parts, the REMS document and associated materials, and the REMS supporting document. "The REMS document establishes the goals and requirements of the REMS [and] describes the elements of the REMS and specific steps for each stakeholder to mitigate the serious risk of the drug," Mehler said. The REMS materials include other documents that FDA has approved for use in meeting the REMS requirements (e.g., certification forms, enrollment forms, educational materials).

The REMS document and materials for all approved REMS are publicly available on the FDA website.[2] Mehler added that the REMS document and materials are enforceable by FDA and cannot be changed without the agency's approval (see REMS modifications, below).

The REMS supporting document is the sponsor's plan for how it will meet the requirement in the REMS document, "and includes the rationale for the design, implementation, and assessment of the REMS," Mehler said. The supporting document is reviewed by FDA during the REMS approval process and when changes are made. REMS supporting documents are not publicly disclosed.

REMS MODIFICATION

The agency or the sponsor can request modifications to the REMS. FDA might suggest that the sponsor consider making a modification, or the agency can issue a formal request for modification via a letter to the sponsor with a specified time period for response, which Mehler said per the statute is "120 days or a reasonable time."

Mehler referred participants to the FDA guidance for industry on REMS modifications and revisions.[3] Editorial revisions that are minor changes to the REMS (e.g., an address change) can be made with notification to FDA. Major modifications to a REMS are changes to the document or materials that are related to product safety or to stakeholder actions required for compliance with the REMS. For example, adding or removing a REMS element or tool is a major change. All major changes must be submitted to FDA as a Prior Approval Supplement and must contain the rationale for the modification, she said. Prior Approval Supplements for major changes are reviewed by FDA within 6 months of receipt by the agency. The statute also includes provisions for dispute resolution if needed, she said.

---

[2] See https://www.accessdata.fda.gov/scripts/cder/rems/index.cfm (accessed November 18, 2023).

[3] See https://www.fda.gov/media/128651/download (accessed November 18, 2023).

OVERLAPPING STATUTORY AUTHORITIES
FOR CONTROLLED SUBSTANCES

Opioids are subject to both controlled substances obligations and REMS obligations. DEA is responsible for implementing controlled substances regulations under the Federal Controlled Substances Act. Controlled substances are also subject to state-controlled substance laws and regulations. Mehler pointed out that for controlled substances, "the DEA statute is the floor," and states can implement additional or more restrictive regulations. FDA is responsible for implementing regulations and guidance under the Federal Food, Drug, and Cosmetic Act, which includes authority to establish product–drug specific obligations via a REMS. By contrast to DEA, FDA regulation preempts state regulation.

DEA statute requires registration of activities and locations that "physically touch the drug," Mehler explained (e.g., manufacturing, warehousing, distribution, dispensing, administering). There is no specific requirement for the drug sponsor to register, and if the sponsor outsources all activities, it is not a DEA registrant, she said. Under FDA regulations, the drug sponsor is always the responsible party for compliance and assessment, regardless of whether it is directly involved in an activity or if the activity is outsourced.

Complying with FDA, DEA, and multiple state regulations can be challenging for sponsors. Mehler said it had long been unclear "where FDA's authority ended and DEA's started" regarding mitigating abuse and the risks associated with diversion. However, since 2008, "REMS authority specifically allows FDA to require a REMS for [adverse events] that are overdose, abuse, and withdrawal," she said.

SUPPORT ACT PROVISIONS

As discussed, FDA's REMS authority was expanded under the SUPPORT Act, giving the agency authority to require interventions (packaging, disposal systems) to mitigate a serious risk. Mehler pointed out that one challenge when developing a REMS is when the risk is associated with a subset of patients or conditions. Language in the law allows FDA to require these interventions "for certain patients." SUPPORT Act provisions also require FDA to consider patient access to the drug, the burden on health care systems, and compatibility with established systems when establishing REMS requirements. In addition, the "agency must consult with other federal agencies with authority over drug disposal packaging," Mehler said.

PRACTICAL CONSIDERATIONS

Mehler discussed the following three categories of practical considerations for implementing opioid disposal systems under a REMS:

- **Will it work?** Considerations listed by Mehler included whether the disposal system meets the DEA standard for rendering the drug unretrievable, whether patients understand how to use it and whether they actually use it, whether it is practical to use across the wide range of settings and conditions where opioids are used, and how to determine which systems are effective and how to regulate these systems.
- **Will it be unduly burdensome?** It is important to consider the potential burdens that use of a disposal system might impose on patients with short-term prescriptions as well as on those taking opioids to manage chronic pain, and how use of the disposal system would impact the health care system, including pharmacies. Mehler also highlighted the need to consider the potential burden for opioid drug manufacturers who must supply the disposal systems (e.g., costs) and whether those burdens might impact their ability to continue to supply the market and meet the opioid product needs of patients.
- **Will there be unintended consequences?** The impact of drug disposal systems on the environment is one potential unintended consequence that has been discussed throughout the workshop. Another consideration is the potential for determined drug seekers to find ways to identify containers with disposed opioids and access them, Mehler said.

6

Regulatory Landscape for Household Opioid Disposal

Highlights of Key Points Made by Individual Speakers*

- The Food and Drug Administration (FDA) has required a risk evaluation and mitigation strategy for all opioid analgesics dispensed in outpatient settings. (Raulerson)
- The recent removal of the non-retrievable standard from the SUPPORT Act allows FDA to consider a wider range of opioid disposal options that could be dispensed to patients. (Raulerson)
- In-home disposal systems can provide an option for people who cannot or do not want to bring their unused drugs to a take-back day or community kiosk. (Dhillon)
- The Environmental Protection Agency (EPA) cannot regulate household hazardous waste disposal, but the agency recommends avoiding disposal of hazardous waste by methods that lead to local landfills. EPA recommends incineration of medication over flushing or landfill disposal. (K. Fitzgerald)
- States and localities may regulate the disposal of household hazardous waste, and some prohibit the disposal of medication in solid waste systems. (Atia, K. Fitzgerald, Kellington)
- Extended producer responsibility laws in some states could present barriers to in-home opioid disposal methods. (Atia)

> *This list is the rapporteurs' summary of points made by the individual speakers identified, and the statements have not been endorsed or verified by the National Academies of Sciences, Engineering, and Medicine. They are not intended to reflect a consensus among workshop participants.

PRODUCT STEWARDSHIP

An overview of product stewardship and extended producer responsibility (EPR) laws was provided by Hanz Atia of PSI. PSI is a non-profit organization that "advocat[es] for sustainable practices and responsible management of the full life cycle of products," working with stakeholders to develop EPR policies, programs, and laws. Atia's work focuses on promoting programs that expand the safe disposal of pharmaceuticals and sharps.

PSI developed the first principles of product stewardship in 2001, Atia said, and the organization's work over the past two decades has led to EPR programs in more than 20 product categories. This includes the passage of 133 EPR laws in 33 states, across 17 product categories.

Atia discussed the following:

- **"Product stewardship** is the act of minimizing the health, safety, environmental, and social impacts of a product and its packaging throughout all life cycle stages while also maximizing economic benefits. Product stewardship can be voluntary or required by law."
- **"Extended producer responsibility** is a mandatory type of product stewardship required by law … [EPR] extends both upstream to product design and downstream to postconsumer reuse, recycling, or safe disposal." Upstream, EPR programs "provid[e] incentives for manufacturers to incorporate environmental considerations in the design of their packaging and products." Downstream, EPR shifts financial and management responsibility from the public sector back to the manufacturer (with government oversight).

Pharmaceutical EPR

PSI began its push to establish convenient drug take-back programs in 2008 by convening stakeholder meetings that called for new laws and regulations. Atia highlighted subsequent legislative and regulatory actions that have led to the passage of 8 state and 23 local pharmaceutical EPR laws to date (Figure 6-1). PSI continues to advocate for and support pharmaceutical EPR programs, creating resources such as briefing documents,

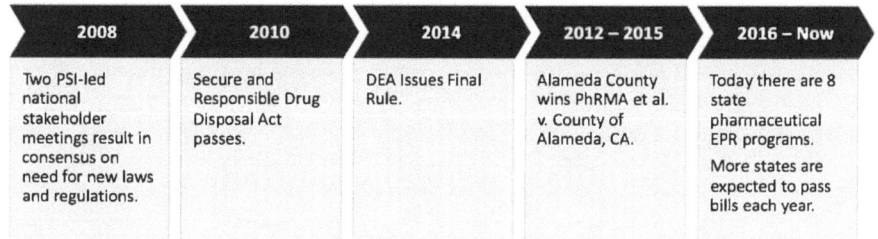

FIGURE 6-1 Timeline of pharmaceuticals stewardship laws.
NOTE: DEA = Drug Enforcement Administration; EPR = extended producer responsibility; PhRMA = Pharmaceutical Research and Manufacturers of America; PSI = Product Stewardship Institute.
SOURCES: Presented by Hanz Atia, June 26, 2023. © Product Stewardship Institute, 2023. Used with permission.

drug take-back pilot demonstrations, a how-to guide for pharmacists,[1] and public and provider educational materials. PSI has also developed a list of "16 elements of an effective EPR law" and helps states to draft model legislation that incorporates EPR best practices, Atia said.

Pharmaceutical EPR laws were first passed by Vermont and Massachusetts in 2016, followed by California, New York, and Washington in 2018, Oregon in 2019, Maine in 2021, and Illinois in 2022. Atia noted that the EPR programs in these eight states are funded by drug manufacturers. They highlighted select elements of the EPR laws in Maine, Illinois, Oregon, and New York that bar, discourage, or present barriers to in-home disposal methods.

Maine

Maine's law specifically excludes in-home disposal methods from stewardship programs, Atia said. Proposed disposal plans

> must ensure that collection methods used under the program include mail-back envelopes and collection receptacles and do not include home disposal methods involving packets, bottles, or other containers that a person may use to render non-retrievable or destroy a covered drug that is household pharmaceutical waste by means of chemical process [Public Law 2021, c. 94, § 2 (NEW)].[2]

---

[1] See https://productstewardship.us/wp-content/uploads/2022/11/160920_PSI_Pharmacy_Guide_vS.pdf (accessed November 18, 2023).

[2] See https://legislature.maine.gov/statutes/38/title38sec1612-1.html (accessed November 18, 2023).

This exclusion appears again later in the law. Atia said this exclusion stems from Maine's experience with active pharmaceutical ingredients in the environment. For example, some organic farms could no longer label products as organic due to the presence of active pharmaceutical ingredients in the water system.

Illinois

The Illinois EPR law has similarities to Maine with regard to in-home disposal. Atia drew attention to a section on promotional materials for a drug take-back program. These materials "may not be used to promote in-home disposal products of any kind including, but not limited to, in-home disposal products of authorized collectors participating in a drug take-back program."[3]

Oregon

Per Oregon law, the operator of the take-back program must "discourage the disposal of covered drugs in the garbage or sewer system."[4]

New York

New York law requires that proposals include "how covered drugs will be safely and securely tracked and handled from collection through final disposal and destruction, [and] policies to ensure security and compliance with all applicable laws and regulations including disposal and destruction at a permitted waste disposal facility meeting federal requirements."[5] Atia said this presents a barrier for in-home disposal systems that are disposed of by patients and are not tracked.

International Approaches

To further inform the discussions, Atia said the European Union EPR program for pharmaceuticals includes drop-off kiosks in pharmacies. In Canada, prescription drugs, OTC medicines, and natural health products are returned to collection sites as part of the Medications Return Program managed and paid for by the Health Product Stewardship Association.

---

[3] See https://www.ilga.gov/legislation/ilcs/ilcs3.asp?ActID=4321&ChapterID=35 (accessed November 18, 2023).

[4] See https://www.oregonlegislature.gov/bills_laws/lawsstatutes/2019orlaw0659.pdf (accessed November 18, 2023).

[5] See https://www.nysenate.gov/legislation/bills/2017/S9100 (accessed November 18, 2023).

In-Home Disposal Compared to Take-Back Programs

In closing, Atia said each of the different drug disposal models has benefits and drawbacks. As discussed, an advantage of in-home systems such as disposal pouches is that they are more accessible for certain populations (e.g., home-bound individuals). However, complexity, cost, environmental impact, and lack of trackability can present challenges.

Regardless of approach, a key element of pharmaceutical EPR programs is a requirement for education and outreach by the manufacturer or program administrator, Atia said. They shared results from a recent survey of 2,000 Americans that found that more than half did not know what to do with unused pharmaceuticals, and more than two-thirds "would be willing to change disposal habits if they knew how."[6]

PERSPECTIVES ON REGULATORY AUTHORITY

Following the presentation, Atia was joined by four panelists who shared their perspectives on the current laws and regulations relevant to in-home drug disposal systems. Panelists included Uttam Dhillon, partner at Michael Best & Friedrich LLP; Kristin Fitzgerald, an environmental protection specialist at EPA; Mary Kellington, Safe Medicine Return program manager for the Washington State Department of Health; and Patrick Raulerson, senior regulatory counsel for CDER at FDA. The discussion was moderated by Lewis Grossman, Ann Loeb Bronfman Professor of Law at American University Washington College of Law.

EPA

Two federal laws implemented by EPA are applicable to the disposal of medication. The Clean Air Act governs incineration, including monitoring and emissions controls, and the Resource Conservation and Recovery Act (RCRA) governs land disposal of hazardous and solid waste, K. Fitzgerald said. RCRA gives EPA regulatory authority over the "cradle-to-grave management of hazardous waste" but excludes household disposal, she explained. States and localities may regulate the disposal of household hazardous waste (e.g., the state pharmaceutical EPR laws discussed by Atia above).

K. Fitzgerald noted that EPA also administers the Clean Water Act and the Safe Drinking Water Act, but neither of these provide authority applicable to in-home drug disposal. EPA can recommend that medica-

---

[6] See https://swnsdigital.com/us/2021/04/more-than-two-thirds-of-americans-dont-know-how-to-properly-dispose-medications-new-research-reveals/ (accessed November 18, 2023).

tions not be flushed, she said, but does not have authority under these laws to prohibit this action. EPA can prohibit flushing of medication by health care facilities under RCRA but has no authority to regulate flushing of medications by households.

EPA is interested in what happens when a product leaves the home—specifically, where it goes and who is exposed to it, K. Fitzgerald said. Again, EPA cannot regulate household disposal, but the agency recommends that people take their hazardous waste (e.g., used motor oil, antifreeze) to household hazardous waste collections and avoid disposal methods that lead to local landfills.

For disposal of unused medication, the consensus recommendation from EPA and all federal agencies is to use pharmaceutical take-back programs (e.g., DEA periodic take-back days or mail-back envelopes, permanent take-back kiosks in the community). "EPA fully supports FDA's recent decision to require manufacturers of opioids to make … prepaid mail-back envelopes available to customers filling opioid prescriptions," K. Fitzgerald said, and EPA looks forward to wider availability of free mail-back envelopes in 2024 (when it is anticipated that the modified REMS will be approved). She explained that mail-back envelopes are destroyed by a "DEA reverse distributor" in a permitted, licensed, controlled incinerator because incineration is currently the only destruction technology that meets the DEA requirement that a disposed controlled substance be non-retrievable. EPA supports this approach, she said, because incineration of mail-back envelopes provides a "dual public health benefit," removing opioids from the home and protecting the environment by reducing the flushing of opioids (which can lead to contamination of sources of drinking water).

The removal of the non-retrievable standard from the SUPPORT Act opens up the possibility for development of in-home disposal kits that could be discarded in household trash. K. Fitzgerald said this approach could mean that pharmaceutical products are still accessible to children, pets, or those seeking drugs until trash pickup day. Furthermore, she said that about 80 percent of trash in the United States goes to landfills (versus incineration), which can lead to pharmaceutical ingredients in the environment. She noted that some in-home disposal kits work mechanistically via adsorption to activated charcoal. However, acidic conditions in landfills can cause desorption and leaching of pharmaceutical ingredients, which are not removed by routine wastewater processing of landfill leachate. Incineration is preferable to landfill disposal because incineration completely destroys the pharmaceutical ingredients, she continued, and leads to a "better environmental outcome" as a result of effective monitoring and emission controls under the Clean Air Act.

FDA

"The opioid analgesic REMS is primarily focused on education of patients and health care practitioners on the safe use of opioids," Raulerson said. FDA has required a REMS for all opioid analgesics dispensed in outpatient settings.

As mentioned, the SUPPORT Act gave FDA the authority to require, as part of a REMS, that certain patients be provided a safe disposal system or disposal packaging with a drug, if it is determined that doing so "could be expected to mitigate the risk of abuse of that drug or overdose associated with that drug, including accidental exposure," Raulerson said. In considering when and how to apply this authority, the agency will consider the potential implications for the health care delivery system. For example, Raulerson said it is important to consider how a REMS modification mandating the provision of disposal systems might impact existing voluntary initiatives (e.g., retail pharmacy disposal programs) and state- and local-level disposal policies and product stewardship programs.

As discussed by Marta Sokolowska, under this new authority FDA is modifying the opioid analgesic REMS to require manufacturers of opioids to make prepaid mail-back envelopes and educational materials available to outpatient dispensers to give patients with their prescribed opioid. The next step will be for the manufacturers to collectively submit a proposal with modifications to the REMS that meet these requirements. FDA will then determine if the proposal is acceptable and approve it. Manufacturers would then begin to implement the changes. He noted that there can be some back and forth on elements of the proposal, and there is a dispute resolution process if needed.

Raulerson said that mail-back envelopes were the first opioid REMS modification mandated because all the necessary systems were already in place. This included the availability of federally regulated incinerators that could be used to meet the DEA requirement that disposed systems be non-retrievable. In addition, he said rules have been in place for a decade that are designed to ensure that mail-back envelopes are fit for purpose.

The removal of the non-retrievable standard from the SUPPORT Act in 2023 "opened the door for [FDA] to consider a wider range of things that might be dispensed to patients," Raulerson said, including the in-home disposal systems that are the subject of this workshop. Raulerson said that, to his knowledge, there is no regulation of in-home drug disposal systems by any federal, state, or local agency to ensure they are fit for purpose. He suggested that minimum specifications and standards for in-home disposal systems would need to be established before FDA would mandate them under a REMS. In this regard, Raulerson said that "this workshop is one of the first places we are having robust discussion of what those specifications might be and how we would create them." There is a range of options for standards development, and the agency is open to discussion. He emphasized that this is new territory, and FDA wants to be sure that rules and standards based on the knowledge and systems of today do not inadvertently stifle innovation or limit the development of better or easier-to-use systems. As discussed throughout the workshop, multiple solutions might be needed to meet the needs of different patients, and he said FDA's primary goal is "removing the risk from the home."

Federal Drug Enforcement

Dhillon shared his perspective as former acting administrator of DEA and a former federal prosecutor. When he joined DEA in 2018, the weight of contributions at each National Prescription Drug Take Back Day that year was nearly 1 million pounds (drugs and packaging). Although this is an important program that gives people an opportunity to return unused drugs, the events only take place twice each year. In addition, he said contributions have declined since 2018 and currently hover around 600,000 pounds for the most recent take-back days. Permanent drop-off kiosks are also available, but use is variable.

A lot of attention is focused on the number of deaths from illicit drug use (e.g., fentanyl, heroin), but the number of people who die from prescription drug overdose is often not discussed, Dhillon said. CDC estimated there were 16,000 overdose deaths involving prescription opioids in 2020, or 44 people each day, he said.[7] Addiction to prescription opioids may lead to fentanyl or heroin misuse and overdose. A significant contributor to this problem is that "prescriptions that are languishing in people's medicine cabinets … are being diverted" and are then used inappropriately. "From a law enforcement perspective, the goal is always to reduce supply," he said.

Dhillon said the simplest way to reduce the supply of diverted prescription drugs (and associated addiction and overdose deaths) is to make it easy for people to eliminate those drugs from their homes. He suggested that in-home disposal is perhaps the easiest method to accomplish that goal. In-home disposal systems provide an option for people who cannot or do not want to bring their unused drugs to a take-back event or community kiosk. Dhillon observed that people can be hesitant to walk into a police station to dispose of drugs.

Participant David Schiller, chief executive officer of NarcX and formerly of DEA, agreed and said the national take-back initiative has been

---

[7] See https://nida.nih.gov/research-topics/trends-statistics/overdose-death-rates (accessed November 18, 2023).

very successful, but some people still perceive an association with criminal activity, and some fear they will be investigated for dropping off unused drugs. Schiller noted that diversion of drugs from the take-back stockpiles prior to destruction is an ongoing concern. Every year there are arrests of law enforcement officers who have stolen drugs from the national take-back or collection kiosks. Schiller emphasized the importance of educating the public about the diversion of unused opioids from homes and the need to dispose.

Washington State: A Case Example of State Regulation of Drug Disposal

Kellington said 26 states now have laws authorizing some kind of drug take-back program. Washington's statewide Safe Medication Return program was launched in 2020 following passage of the state's drug take-back law in 2018. Kellington explained that the state law was modeled after successful local ordinances, and that existing local take-back programs were incorporated into the state program.

"Safe Medication Return accepts prescription and over-the-counter medications in any dose and in any form," Kellington said, including pet medications. Medical devices containing drugs are accepted, but empty medical devices, exposed needles, and sharps are not. Also excluded are "vitamins, homeopathic remedies, schedule 1 drugs, and drugs administered in a clinical setting."

Products can be returned using free prepaid mailers (ordered online or by phone or picked up at one of 442 mailer distribution locations in the community); deposited at one of 800 widely distributed secure collection kiosks (e.g., pharmacies, law enforcement agencies, long-term care facilities, and substance use disorder treatment programs); or brought to community take-back events. Kellington noted that only 2 of the state's 281 population centers do not have return kiosks or mailer distribution sites, and mailers are distributed in these areas via direct mail campaigns. All products collected are incinerated, and the program costs are covered by drug manufacturers, she said. More than 175 tons of product have been collected by Safe Medication Return since inception. Kellington said that although less than 2 percent of returned medication is given back via mail, the mailers are an important option and provide access for residents who are not served by or do not want to use kiosks and/or collection events.

Kellington said nothing in Washington state law prohibits the use of other in-home disposal methods, but she believed it was "unlikely" that methods other than mailers could be incorporated into the state-regulated program. She also pointed out that some local ordinances prohibit the disposal of medication at solid waste facilities (e.g., King County's Waste

Acceptance Rule[8]). Safe Medication Return program operators are also required by the take-back law to discourage people from flushing medication or placing it in the trash.

---

[8] See https://kingcounty.gov/en/legacy/about/policies/rules/utilities/put716pr (accessed November 18, 2023).

7

Scientific Considerations for In-Home Opioid Disposal

Highlights of Key Points Made by Individual Speakers*

- Ideally, an in-home opioid disposal system would be non-toxic and non-hazardous; render active pharmaceutical ingredients unusable; deter misuse; and limit environmental contamination. (Coop, Horwitz)
- Performance questions for in-home disposal systems include whether a system is safe for the user, renders drugs undesirable, renders drugs non-retrievable, and is safe to dispose of in a solid waste system after addition of drugs. (Shield)
- Performance testing of disposal systems is generally done one drug at a time, but in real-world settings, people are likely to dispose of multiple different drugs and dosage forms together. (Shield, Wood)
- Efficacy of disposal systems should be assessed using actual dosage forms, not just pure active pharmaceutical ingredients. (Coop, Shield)
- Ideally, the packaging of in-home disposal systems would be child-resistant and have labeling that clearly explains both the time needed for full inactivation of the drug as well as the need to securely store the product–drug mixture until that point and discard it promptly after that point. (Brown, Shield)
- Regulatory agencies would need to know the components of a drug disposal system to evaluate the effectiveness of the

49

system for rendering a drug unusable and assessing toxicity. (Coop)
- For transparency, regulatory agencies could require that drug disposal systems be analyzed by independent laboratories, including a waste determination assessment, with full disclosure results. (Shield)
- It would be necessary to know the components of a drug disposal system to test the effectiveness of the system in preventing the environmental release of drugs. (Bradley)

*This list is the rapporteurs' summary of points made by the individual speakers identified, and the statements have not been endorsed or verified by the National Academies of Sciences, Engineering, and Medicine. They are not intended to reflect a consensus among workshop participants.

ASSESSING UTILITY AND PERFORMANCE

Margaret Shield, a public health and environment health consultant and owner and principal of Community Environmental Health Strategies LLC, provided background on assessing the utility and performance of medication disposal systems. The safe and environmentally responsible disposal of medicines "reduces availability for misuse, addiction, and overdose; helps prevent unintended poisonings; [and] prevents pollution from waste medicines," she said. Shield emphasized that these three issues are interconnected, and developing solutions for one without considering how those solutions affect the others could lead to unintended consequences.

Shield based her remarks on the March 2019 report *Medicine Disposal Products: An Overview of Products and Performance Questions* that her company prepared for the San Francisco Department of the Environment.[1] The report reviewed medicine disposal systems available at the time and sought to answer four main questions about system safety and performance (Box 7-1). Shield noted that there are no plans to update the 2019 report and added that "it should not fall on local government budgets to review or test these products."

---

[1] See https://sfenvironment.org/sites/default/files/fliers/files/medicinedisposalproducts_march2019.pdf (accessed November 18, 2023).

> **BOX 7-1**
> **Key Performance Questions for Disposal Systems Assessed in the 2019 Report on In-Home Disposal Systems**
>
> Is the disposal system safe for the user?
> - "Are product ingredients safe?
> - Does the product as sold contain any hazardous chemicals?
> - Are users protected from exposure to active pharmaceuticals when using the product?
> - Are instructions easy to follow and warning labels complete?"
>
> Does the disposal system render the drugs undesirable?
> - "Does the product act as a deterrent for medicine abuse or accidental ingestion?
> - Are medicines disguised or made physically inaccessible?
> - Are medicines made unpalatable for ingestion?"
>
> Does the disposal system render the drugs non-retrievable?
> - "Are medicines recoverable from the product mixture?
> - Are pharmaceuticals permanently physically or chemically altered?
> - Does the product's action meet the Drug Enforcement Administration's non-retrievable standard for disposal of controlled substances?"
>
> Is the combined product–drug mixture safe for solid waste disposal?
> - "Is the product–drug mixture in solid or liquid form?
> - Can the product–drug mixture be released in the garbage can or compactor truck?
> - Is the product–drug mixture toxic or otherwise hazardous?
> - Does the product–drug mixture meet federal, Tribal, state, and local requirements for solid waste disposal?"
>
> SOURCE: Presented by Margaret Shield, June 26, 2023, citing the March 2019 report by Community Environmental Health Strategies LLC.

Key Performance Questions

Is the Disposal System Safe for the User?

For the disposal systems available at the time of the review, Shield found that assessment of safety was a challenge as ingredients were often not fully disclosed. Examples of ingredients listed included activated carbon, bentonite clay (an ingredient of kitty litter), and calcium hypochlorite (a concentrated, solid form of chlorine and a powerful oxidizer), as well as non-descript ingredients such as "denaturing agents" and "organic plant-based powder." Some systems had strong chemical odors. She noted that the use of child-resistant packaging by disposal systems was variable.

Disposal systems required dissolving the drug in water or unknown solvents that were provided. Shield found that there was a potential for spills from pouch-type disposal systems, and some product labels warned of the potential for foaming or release of gas, but there were no label warnings regarding the safety of the resulting product–drug mixture for exposed skin and no clean-up instructions for spills.

Shield offered several recommendations to address some of the user safety concerns identified in the report. These included

- improving labeling to clarify non-specific and confusing instructions (e.g., "not for use with drugs known to react with each other") and to warn users to avoid skin contact with contents;
- listing all product ingredients and identifying those that are hazardous;
- addressing the potential for leakage (e.g., by adding absorbents or solidifying agents) and including instructions for cleaning up spills; and
- using child-resistant packaging.

Does the Disposal System Render the Drugs Undesirable?

Shield found that "deterrence impact does vary by product." She suggested that the noxious nature of some system ingredients might make them less desirable for misuse. Other systems state their ingredients are "plant-based" or safe for use in food, which could be interpreted as edible. She also observed that when ready for disposal in the trash, all but one of the systems had labels that clearly indicated there was medication inside, making it easy for someone seeking drugs to find it.

Does the Disposal System Render the Drugs Non-Retrievable?[2]

Data on testing for retrievability of disposed drugs were not available for all systems assessed in the 2019 review at the time of publication, Shield said. Some systems advertise that they "deactivate," "destroy," or "degrade" drugs, but laboratory testing results available in 2019 indicate that some active pharmaceutical ingredient is still retrievable. Other available testing indicated that washing the product–drug mixture with water was sufficient to desorb some of the drug from an activated charcoal dis-

---

[2] The non-retrievable requirement was removed from the SUPPORT Act in the Consolidated Appropriations Act of 2023.

posal system. Shield also noted that complete adsorption of the drug to be disposed can take several hours to several days, and adsorption is impacted by chemical properties of the drug (e.g., solubility). Importantly, testing of disposal systems for non-retrievability was generally done for a small quantity of an individual drug. Actual consumers are likely to use the system to dispose of a combination of different drugs, and types of drugs, at once.

Summarizing her findings from the 2019 review, Shield said that "overall, the available testing data [were] not convincing that any of the systems demonstrated irreversible physical or chemical destruction of controlled substances."

Is the Combined Product–Drug Mixture Safe for Solid Waste Disposal?

Various concerns regarding disposal in the solid waste system are discussed in the 2019 report. The product–drug mixture for disposal could be "in liquid or slurry or wet gel form," and "liquid waste is typically not accepted in the garbage or in landfills," Shield said. The packaging containing the product–drug mixture is subject to damage in the trash can or garbage truck, resulting in leaks (which Shield pointed out could occur before the drug has been fully adsorbed/becomes non-retrievable). In 2019, the resulting product–drug mixtures had not been fully characterized as non-hazardous and non-toxic, she continued. Drug disposal systems might be labeled as safe for trash disposal, but the burden is on residents to determine if local solid waste regulations permit disposal in their trash. Furthermore, local regulators might find it challenging to assess the acceptability of these systems for solid waste disposal given the limited information available about their ingredients, mechanisms of action, and performance, she said.

Performance Testing and Regulatory Oversight of In-Home Opioid Disposal Systems

Shield shared her recommendations on performance testing of drug disposal systems that are discussed in the 2019 report. She said these recommendations are relevant to in-home opioid disposal systems and would be "the minimum basic analysis that FDA needs to assess the utility and impacts of these products."

- "Require independent laboratory analysis and full disclosure of analytical reports."
- "Test drug mixtures [and] combinations of different dosage forms to better represent 'real world' consumer use. Consumers generally do not just dispose of opioids."

- "Use appropriate analytic designs to assess deterrence and to assess non-retrievability of pharmaceuticals."
- "Conduct complete waste determination of the product with treated drugs to assess if appropriate for solid waste disposal. A variety of tests will be required to assess compliance with diverse state, local, and Tribal regulations."

Shield also emphasized the need for appropriate regulatory oversight and enforcement authority, reiterating the point by Patrick Raulerson that consumer drug disposal systems are currently unregulated. Monitoring is needed to ensure consumer safety and system performance relative to what is claimed. In addition, "any new federal regulatory structure needs to respect local authority for waste management practices," she said. In this regard, Shield emphasized the need to engage "local solid waste agenc[y], local wastewater, local public health, [and] local law enforcement" professionals who have been working for many years to provide safe drug disposal options that meet the needs of their communities. She observed that there was a lack of local expertise represented at the workshop and said these technical and regulatory experts from local agencies "can help define the analysis that is needed to fully evaluate these medicine disposal products."

In addition to the four key performance questions for disposal systems previously discussed, Shield suggested that in-home opioid disposal systems be evaluated relative to take-back programs as a standard. Specifically, she proposed the following questions for assessment of in-home opioid disposal systems before implementation in a REMS:

- "Is it a better solution for residents than a comprehensive drug take-back program?"[3]
- Who should use it? (e.g., everyone or primarily those unable to use an available drug take-back option).
- "For what drugs and dosage forms?" (e.g., all drugs or only opioids; pills, patches, liquids).
- Will it complement or interfere with "the convenient, safe and secure, and environmentally sound drug take-back programs that are already operating?"
- Will public messaging align with or conflict with recommendations from state and local governments and community groups to bring unused drugs to local drug take-back programs?

---

[3] Shield clarified that a comprehensive drug take-back program incorporates "pharmacy-based drop boxes, prepaid return mailers on demand, and periodic collection events" that are free to consumers and equitably distributed. Unified opioid education and promotion of take-back services are also essential elements of a comprehensive plan.

In closing, Shield referred participants to model pharmaceutical stewardship legislation she helped develop that can serve as a guide for state policy makers. She also suggested that an action FDA could take now would be to modify the current opioid REMS to "require opioid manufacturers to fund and operate a public-friendly website and toll-free number to connect residents in every state with all available drug take-back services in their area."

SCIENTIFIC CONSIDERATIONS

Following the presentation, Shield was joined by four panelists for a discussion of the ideal characteristics of an in-home drug disposal system from mechanistic, safety, and environmental perspectives, and approaches for assessing the environmental impact of such systems. Panelists included Paul Bradley, project lead in the Drinking-Water and Wastewater Infrastructure Integrated Science Team in the Ecosystems Mission, Environmental Health Program, at the U.S. Geological Survey; Kaitlyn Brown, clinical managing director for America's Poison Centers; Andrew Coop, professor of pharmaceutical sciences and an associate dean for academic affairs at the University of Maryland School of Pharmacy; and Marta Sokolowska. The discussion was moderated by Jessica Young, chief of the Recycling and Generator Branch in the Office of Resource Conservation and Recovery at EPA.

Exposure Data from the National Poison Data System

Exposures to In-Home Drug Disposal Systems

America's Poison Centers represents 55 poison centers across the United States and maintains the National Poison Data System, a near real-time poisoning data repository.[4] Brown said the repository does have some data on exposures to in-home disposal systems. She noted that data collection is hampered by the fact that registration of disposal systems is voluntary. Therefore, not all available disposal kits that people might call in to report are in the product database for the poison specialists to select. Broad registration of disposal systems in the poison database would better enable tracking of exposures and outcomes, she said.

Of the disposal systems that are listed in the database, more than 200 exposures have been reported since 2019. Sixty percent of these reported exposures have been in adults, and most are accidental exposure to the

---

[4] See https://www.aapcc.org/national-poison-data-system (accessed November 18, 2023).

disposal system itself. For most of the cases the route of exposure is ingestion, but there are also thermal and ocular exposures, and an individual might report multiple routes of exposure. "Most cases are resulting in no effect or only minimally bothersome symptoms," Brown said. Although about 15 percent sought medical attention, there were no significant effects or deaths.

Pediatric Opioid Exposure Data

Brown also provided a brief overview of registry data on pediatric opioid exposures. She said that reports of pediatric opioid exposure to poison centers declined from 2019 to June 2023. One possible explanation for this decline, she suggested, is that increased awareness about opioids might be motivating parents to take their child directly to a hospital rather than calling a poison center for advice. Another possibility is that health care providers are now more informed about opioid exposures and are less likely to consult a poison center for guidance. She noted that voluntary reporting is a limitation of the poison center data.

Although overall exposure reports have declined, the different types of opioid drugs involved in accidental pediatric exposures have expanded. Buprenorphine is the most common opioid exposure in children from birth to age 5, Brown said, "followed by oxycodone alone or in combination [and] hydrocodone alone or in combination with other products." She added that accidental exposure in young children is generally "exploratory ingestion" of drugs they encounter in their environment. Of the more than 3,100 accidental exposures in this age group in 2022, 80 percent sought medical attention, and "10 percent of those cases resulted in a major effect or death," Brown said.

Efficacy Considerations for Drug Disposal Systems

To test the effectiveness of drug disposal systems in preventing the environmental release of drugs, it would be necessary to know the components of the system, Bradley said. Then it might be possible to identify a tracer to detect signals in the water environment. However, nothing in current disposal systems allows for detection in the environment.

Coop acknowledged that companies are unlikely to release proprietary information about specific components of their disposal systems (e.g., exactly what their "cross-linking polymer" is). He suggested following a model like that used for tobacco products, in which manufacturers make their ingredients known to FDA. Without knowing what the components are, it is not possible to determine their toxicity or their efficacy in making the drug unusable. Ultimately, "nothing is ever completely non-retrievable," Coop said. But perhaps it could be difficult enough to retrieve to deter attempts. He likened this approach to the development of abuse-deterrent formulations for opioids.

Shield agreed and said her review of the available testing data raised many additional questions. She reiterated that disposal system testing is generally done one drug at a time, when in real-world use people are likely to dispose of multiple drugs in one disposal system. "Drugs have different hydrophobic and hydrophilic properties," she said. Some are not readily dissolvable, which she said was noted in some testing results she reviewed. In some cases, it was not clear if the testing of disposal systems could distinguish between when a drug was adsorbed to the charcoal and when it was simply not in solution. She highlighted the need for testing of drug disposal systems to be done by accredited laboratories using appropriate controls. Her review found that pure active pharmaceutical ingredient was frequently used as a control for the testing. The most appropriate control, however, would be the actual dosage form of the drug (i.e., the active pharmaceutical ingredient and excipient components). Coop added that the active pharmaceutical ingredients are usually in powder form, but opioids can be in abuse-deterrent formulations that are specifically designed to prevent isolation of the active pharmaceutical ingredient. He agreed with the importance of looking at efficacy of disposal systems with the actual dosage forms (e.g., capsule, tablet, liquid, patch) and not just the active pharmaceutical ingredient. Sokolowska noted that the vast majority of opioids currently found in homes are not in abuse-deterrent formulations.

Alastair Wood agreed that it is unlikely consumers will only use disposal systems for removing opioids from the home. He pointed out that it is not possible to conduct safety and performance testing of disposal systems for all possible combinations of drugs that might be disposed along with opioids. Coop said activated charcoal is effective for adsorption of drugs because it has a large surface area per weight[5] and has long been used to adsorb ingested drugs. He suggested that the use of activated charcoal could be highly effective for disposing of multiple drugs if there were a way to immobilize the drug-carbon complex and prevent desorption. Shield added that "consumers are not chemists," so it would be challenging to develop chemical methods "that people can do in their kitchens that would successfully denature or degrade all the different medicines that we use in our homes."

Given the scientific challenges discussed, Shield urged FDA to consider a range of drug disposal options for opioids. Sokolowska agreed

---

[5] Coop clarified that adsorption is when one component sticks to the surface of another. Absorption is when one component soaks into the other.

that a "multipronged" approach is needed to be able to reach all patients with drugs in the home. Sokolowska said FDA "strongly support[s]" the range of efforts being undertaken to remove unused opioids from the home, including take-back days, disposal kiosks, and mail-back envelopes. Yet, more than half of unused opioid prescriptions are still in patients' homes. The task at hand is to understand why people are not discarding these drugs and find ways to better educate and motivate people to remove them from their homes. In doing so, she said it is important not to let perfect be the enemy of good. She suggested that the removal of the non-retrievable standard from the SUPPORT Act by the Consolidated Appropriations Act was done in "recogni[tion] that leaving opioids in homes is a greater risk than removing them with less than perfect options."

Shield also suggested looking to pharmacy-based drug return programs in other countries as models. These are long-standing programs, she said, while pharmacy take-back of controlled substances in the United States has only been allowed under DEA regulation since 2014. She mentioned the Cyclamed take-back program in France as an example, which she said has high rates of return.[6] Sokolowska agreed there are lessons to be learned from regulatory authorities in other countries. However, the ability to implement similar models could be impacted by differences in regulatory frameworks and payment structures between the United States and other countries.

Minimum Requirements for In-Home Opioid Disposal Systems

Participants discussed minimum requirements for an in-home disposal system from a scientific perspective. Coop said an in-home disposal system should ideally be non-toxic. "We cannot have the solution worse than the problem," he said. Still, people are used to using bleach in their homes and calcium hypochlorite is similar. If it were to be used, there would need to be safety education for users (lest they inadvertently create chlorine gas). He also reiterated the need for all components of disposal systems to be identified.

Brown called for minimum packaging standards that could reduce the occurrence of inadvertent exposures to both the disposal system and the product–drug mixture. This would include child-resistant closures and "clear, non-deceptive labeling," she said. For example, users need to understand how long it will take for the drug to be fully inactivated after adding it to the disposal system, and that some drug could still be accessible and pose a risk until that point. Labeling should also emphasize that

---

[6] See https://www.cyclamed.org/english/ (accessed November 18, 2023).

the used system that then contains the drug should be kept secure until it can be properly disposed of, Brown said, and that it should be disposed of promptly and not be retained in the home.

Shield agreed that understanding the timing of inactivation of the disposed drug is important, especially if systems are reaching the landfill before inactivation is complete. She also raised the issue of package integrity for product–drug mixtures that are in liquid form. She noted that disposal systems in the form of resealable plastic bags or plastic bottles are likely to break open in the trash before reaching the landfill. Furthermore, as discussed, local solid waste regulations might prohibit disposal of liquid waste in the trash. She suggested that a solidifying agent might be added after an appropriate time for deactivation. Young added that liquid in disposal systems can leach out over time in landfills and contaminate the environment.

Shield also said that two disposal systems reviewed in her report were designed to be used until full, and the label listed the number of solid form dosages the bottle could contain. She raised concerns about where in the home one would keep this disposal system, which would be partially filled with disposed drugs mixed in some liquid or other medium.

Echoing Sokolowska, Jeff Horwitz said, "We cannot wait for perfection." Opioids in the home are a known risk to people and to the environment. Horwitz summarized what he perceived from the discussions as the main takeaway points on minimal criteria for in-home opioid disposal kits. The disposal system should "change the physical integrity of the drug," "render the active ingredients unusable to mitigate the risk of non-medical use or overdose," "be non-toxic and non-hazardous or pose no threat to the consumer and reduce drug exposure to the environment," and "be a deterrent to … misuse [of the drug]." Coop agreed and said rendering the drug unusable will help stem the diversion of opioids. Coop added that there is a need for disposal systems to address the issue of leaching into the environment.

8

Real-World Implementation and Use of In-Home Opioid Disposal Systems

> **Highlights of Key Points Made by Individual Speakers***
> - Ease of disposal is a key motivating factor for both patients and providers. (Brummett, Shamp, Tsatoke)
> - Qualitative studies suggest that willingness to dispose is influenced more by convenience than by financial incentives. Ensuring the safety of household members is also a motivator. (Brummett)
> - Some reasons for not disposing of unused opioids include lack of awareness, inconvenience of disposal, anticipated future need, and being unable or unwilling to bring drugs to a take-back site (especially a site within a law enforcement facility). (Brummett)
> - Randomized controlled trials and pilot programs have demonstrated that providing an in-home disposal kit increases disposal behavior. (Brummett, Tsatoke)
> - Information about the safe and effective use of in-home disposal systems should be clear, concise, and actionable, and communicated by a trusted source. Contradictory messaging and presentation of uncertain information as fact can undermine public trust. (Krishnamurti)
> - Communications and behavioral interventions should be developed by interdisciplinary teams and include people with relevant lived experience from the start. Interven-

tions should then be pretested before implementation. (Krishnamurti)
- There are multiple touchpoints along the patient care pathway that may offer opportunities for communication about in-home disposal and could also be leveraged to evaluate how a particular intervention might improve uptake of opioid disposal. (Brummett, Krishnamurti, Lewis, Tsatoke)
- State-level programs that provide broad access to drug disposal options can serve as models for the Food and Drug Administration when considering risk evaluation and mitigation strategy (REMS) modifications. (Nicholson)
- Challenges for implementing REMS modifications are communicating the updated requirements, motivating the desired behaviors, and assessing the efficacy of the mitigation strategy. (Shamp)

*This list is the rapporteurs' summary of points made by the individual speakers identified, and the statements have not been endorsed or verified by the National Academies of Sciences, Engineering, and Medicine. They are not intended to reflect a consensus among workshop participants.

OPPORTUNITIES AND BARRIERS FOR THE DISPOSAL OF UNUSED OPIOIDS

Chad Brummett, the Bert N. LaDu Professor of Anesthesiology, co-director of the Opioid Prescribing Engagement Network (OPEN), and co-director of the Opioid Research Institute at the University of Michigan Medical School, set the context for his presentation by sharing the story of a friend, Becky Savage, a nurse and mother of four boys. Her son Jack had just graduated from high school and her son Nick had recently finished his freshman year at college. Someone brought a bottle of pills to a graduation party that Jack and Nick attended together, and both young men "took the pills, drank a couple of beers, and went home, had dinner, and went to bed," Brummett said. The next morning Savage found her two oldest sons were dead. In memory of her sons, Savage established the 525 Foundation, which is committed to raising awareness about the risks of prescription drug misuse.[1] The organization also holds take-back days and has installed secure disposal drop boxes in the Northern

---

[1] See https://www.525foundation.org (accessed November 18, 2023).

Indiana region (19 thus far), which Brummett said have collected more than 50,000 pounds of drugs in about 6 years.

A 2017 systematic review found that 60 to 90 percent of the patients in the included studies reported having unused opioids after surgery (Bicket et al., 2017). He acknowledged that there have been efforts to reduce acute care prescribing in recent years while still ensuring the patient's pain is sufficiently managed. Brummett added that prescribing of opioids to children continues, particularly in association with dental procedures, and opioids that are misused by children ages 12 and older are frequently those that were prescribed for their own care. He suggested that a future National Academies workshop might consider how to reduce opioid prescribing to children, particularly by dentists.

When his group held its first opioid take-back drive in 2016 in Ann Arbor, Michigan, Brummett said it was done as a service to the community and a way to raise awareness of the risks of unused opioids. However, the events also unexpectedly provided data as residents were asked if they would share how they obtained the opioid they were disposing. The most common reason the opioids had been prescribed was for acute care such as surgery, dentistry, or emergency medicine, he said. Less than 20 percent were prescribed the opioid for chronic pain (23 percent could not recall). Since then, OPEN has launched a take-back toolkit (discussed below) and more than 100 sites in 46 counties across the state have participated in a take-back event, netting 28,000 pounds of unused medications. Brummett shared that the oldest drug collected was from 1975, and medications from the 1970s, 1980s, and 1990s are not uncommon.

Studies of Disposal Behaviors

Brummett described an RCT he conducted on the effect of providing an activated charcoal bag for in-home opioid disposal following outpatient surgery. About 25 percent of patients who received usual care and about 30 percent of those who were given an educational information sheet about disposal self-reported having disposed of unused opioids, compared with about 60 percent of those who were given an activated charcoal in-home disposal bag (Brummett et al., 2019).[2] Similar results were found by other RCTs testing postsurgical provision of in-home disposal systems. In a study of pediatric patients, Lawrence and colleagues (2019) found that about 72 percent of parents provided with an in-home disposal bag self-reported disposing of unused opioid versus about 56 percent in the control group. Agarwal and colleagues (2022) found that

---

[2] Patients were given a Deterra Drug Deactivation System. Brummett said he has no financial interest in the Deterra system.

60 percent of patients given in-home disposal bags self-reported having disposed of unused drug versus about 43 percent of those in the control group. However, a study by Bicket and colleagues (2021) found that only 14 percent of participants given an in-home disposal bag reported using it, versus 10 percent of those in the control group. Brummett said a meta-analysis of the RCTs is planned.

Brummett and colleagues are working to understand why people do or do not dispose of unused opioids. In a survey by the National Poll on Healthy Aging, 86 percent of respondents ages 50 to 80 said they saved leftover opioids for later use. Nine percent said they disposed of them in the trash or by flushing, and 13 percent brought them to a take-back location (Harbaugh et al., 2020). Brummett said that early on, "about 80 percent of the safe disposal sites in the state of Michigan were [at] law enforcement [facilities]." Anecdotally, people have reported not wanting to take unused medications to a police station, and some have gone but left without leaving their medications, saying they felt like a criminal, Brummett said.

Studies have also assessed the impact of financial incentives on disposal behavior. In one qualitative study, responses indicated that convenience had a greater influence than financial incentives on willingness to dispose (Draper et al., 2022). Brummett summarized that "making it easy … less than 5 minutes to do it, was more important than giving people $50."

The qualitative study by Draper and colleagues and another by Huang and colleagues looked at facilitators and barriers of disposal, and Brummett summarized themes from the findings (Draper et al., 2022; Huang et al., 2023). Facilitators identified included "convenience; financial incentives; safety of family members; moral beliefs; risk of addiction; risk of theft; [and] risk of environmental harms." Barriers identified included "lack of awareness; less convenient method or process; smaller financial incentive; anticipation of future pain; perception of opioid scarcity; desire to misuse opioids; low perceived risk; [and] breakdown of patient/provider relationship."

Further studies are needed, Brummett said, to identify effective disposal tools and effective ways to influence or incentivize disposal behavior, and he suggested looking to the field of behavioral economics.

Resources and Initiatives from a Community Network

In closing, Brummett referred participants to Michigan's OPEN initiative, which has educational resources that are free to anyone, including materials about the safe disposal of opioids, sharps, and liquids.[3] OPEN

---

[3] See https://michigan-open.org (accessed November 18, 2023).

will also insert a practice's or health system's logo on the front page of the materials for their use, and Brummett said there are "several hundred health systems around the country using our materials." There is a toolkit for setting up a local opioid take-back event and a guide for implementing a permanent disposal box, and OPEN staff are available to provide guidance and support.

In addition to safe disposal, OPEN is working to promote appropriate opioid prescribing while ensuring pain management needs are met for surgical, dental, and emergency medicine patients. Other initiatives focus on ethical approaches to screening patients for substance use disorders and transitioning patients to care; statewide distribution of naloxone; provider, patient, and community education; and informing policy making.

REAL-WORLD EXPERIENCE

Following the presentation, Brummett was joined by five panelists for a discussion of the issues surrounding the implementation and use of in-home opioid disposal systems in real-world settings. Panelists included Tamar Krishnamurti, assistant professor of medicine and clinical and translational science in the Department of Medicine Center for Research on Health Care at the University of Pittsburgh; Eleanor T. Lewis, deputy director of the Program Evaluation and Resource Center at the U.S. Department of Veterans Affairs (VA); Kevin Nicholson, vice president of public policy, regulatory, and legal affairs at the National Association of Chain Drug Stores (NACDS); James Shamp, vice president for data intelligence and program analytics at United BioSource LLC; and CDR Andrea Tsatoke, injury prevention specialist, IHS Headquarters. The discussion was moderated by Mark Bicket, assistant professor, director, pain & opioid research, Department of Anesthesiology, Institute for Healthcare Policy and Innovation at the University of Michigan Medical School.

Providing Multiple Opioid Disposal Options to Meet Patient Needs

Nicholson shared the retail pharmacy perspective on disposal of unused opioids, speaking on behalf of NACDS. "Providing the public with numerous disposal options can help to reduce the unused opioid medications that might otherwise sit in the patient's medicine cabinet," Nicholson said. He described the recent REMS modification on mail-back envelopes as "a good first step in improving access to drug disposal tools" and said NACDS "encourage[s] FDA to further leverage its REMS authorities to expand drug disposal offerings available to the public to include in-home disposal systems." Brummett agreed and said, "Multiple options are critical."

As discussed, several states have successfully implemented programs that provide broad access to drug disposal options, and Nicholson suggested that these state programs can serve as models for FDA. He highlighted the Iowa program through which residents can get two free disposal kits per month (pharmacies are reimbursed for the kits dispensed and associated patient education).

NACDS is submitting comments on in-home disposal options to FDA via the public docket. Nicholson summarized some of the organization's suggestions for modifications to the opioid analgesic REMS, such as requiring "manufacturers to continue to fund and provide disposal options," including pharmacies, among the stakeholders authorized to offer these disposal options to consumers, and reimbursing pharmacies for providing kits and associated services. Furthermore, Nicholson said disposal kits should not be dispensed automatically but rather "should be provided upon patient request." Dispensing of a drug disposal system should follow a conversation "at the point of prescribing or at the point of dispensing" so that patients are aware of the disposal options available to them and can choose which option best meets their needs, he said.

Pilot Distribution Program Experience

Tsatoke said that opioid-related emergency department visits, hospitalizations, and deaths have risen sharply among American Indians and Alaska Natives in recent years, particularly in Arizona. Qualitative data from surveys, interviews, and focus groups revealed that opioid medications were not being properly disposed and there was theft and diversion of unsecured prescriptions. IHS staff conducting home assessments have also found that some patients are stockpiling medication, often unsecured. Anecdotal information provided by pharmacies and law enforcement indicated there is a lack of awareness and education about how to dispose of medications.

To address these concerns, IHS conducted a pilot project to evaluate whether distribution of disposal bags was feasible and effective for the Tribal communities the agency serves (Tsatoke et al., 2021). Tsatoke said planning began by securing Tribal approvals and then meeting with partners in pharmacies and behavioral health as well as public health nurses and community health representatives. She explained that community health representatives are trusted members of the community who are trained as home health aides.

The pilot program was conducted in five Arizona Tribal communities, both urban and very rural. Tsatoke said the pilot was successful, with in-home drug disposal bags distributed to 162 households, resulting in collection of more than 8,000 pills as well as some medicated patches and liquid medication. This in-home disposal option was believed to have complemented other approaches being implemented and evaluated (e.g., secure collection sites and medication lockboxes for safe in-home storage).

REMS Implementation Challenges

Shamp discussed what he said are the two biggest challenges for implementation of a modified REMS, communicating the changes and motivating the desired behaviors. He explained that REMS communication plans have not changed since FDA was first granted REMS authority in 2007. REMS requirements are disseminated via email and U.S. mail, and through outreach to professional societies. Based on his nearly two decades of experience in REMS design and implementation, he said that "that type of communication does not work," and letters frequently go unopened. Clinicians now consume information on smart phones and devices, he said. Communication methods to reach patients must consider the intended audience, he said. For example, he said his 80-year-old mother and his 34-year-old son would both need to receive the same information, but the method would need to be tailored to how they consume information, which is quite different. For all audiences, communications need to be timely and meaningful to recipients, providing specific information so they understand what actions need to be taken, Shamp said.

With regard to motivating prescribers in response to REMS communications, Shamp said, "You typically do not get the behavior you are expecting until it is absolutely necessary, until someone hits a pain point." As an example, he said that providers must become certified and enrolled to prescribe a drug with a REMS. In his experience, he said providers generally do not take these steps until a patient presents in the office in need of the drug. The challenge is how to motivate the necessary prescriber actions before the patient is in need.

There can also be patient requirements in REMS. For example, Shamp said some REMS require that patients have laboratory tests done before receiving a prescription for the drug, as well as after completion of treatment. In such cases, the motivation to have the testing done before prescribing is high. But there is no motivation to do the posttreatment testing, he said, and there can be disincentives, such as co-payments or the need to take action such as driving to the testing site. The challenge for opioids is also motivating patients to take an action after completion of treatment (in this case, destroying the drug).

Lewis also discussed the need to motivate patients to dispose, whether using existing options or increasing the number of options available to them.[4] She said that "even when patients are motivated to dispose of extra medications, there may be barriers to engaging in safe disposal using the primary available options." As discussed, people retain unused opioids for a host of reasons, from the sense of security they get from having the drug "just in case," to practical reasons such as the inconvenience or inaccessibility of a prescriber or a pharmacy, or the cost of a refill.

Shamp added that a key element of REMS implementation is assessment of the efficacy of the mitigation, and it will be necessary to determine how to measure whether in-home disposal systems are effective.

Elements of Effective Consumer Communications

Krishnamurti discussed developing effective consumer communications on safe and effective use of in-home disposal systems from a behavioral science perspective. As has been mentioned, "communications need to be both accessible and actionable," she said. They need to first reach the target audience, and then provide the information needed for making decisions and taking action. Actionable messaging must consider the different ways people will perceive the risks and benefits of acting given their situation (e.g., perceptions of the risks and benefits of retaining unused opioids by someone who has had oral surgery will likely differ from those of someone who has cancer).

Explaining why specific actions are recommended is also important. To illustrate, Krishnamurti shared an anecdote in which she asked three people why mixing pills into kitty litter was recommended prior to discarding. Responses were (1) as a deterrent to those who might ingest them, (2) to neutralize environmental impacts when disposed, and (3) to mask them in the trash. If the person who thought it was a neutralizer does not happen to have kitty litter, that person might decide to retain the opioids, not knowing of any alternative substance to use. The person who thought it was to mask appearance might use a similar substance that achieves the same masking result. "If someone is just not sure why they are being asked to do something, the easiest thing is to do nothing at all," she said.

Information communicated should be clear and concise and be delivered by a trusted source, Krishnamurti continued. She noted that doctors are generally a trusted source, but as discussed, patients can be overwhelmed with the volume of information they receive in a health care encounter, even more so when under the stress of discussing a serious health situation. She also highlighted the need to be transparent about any uncertainties regarding the interventions being implemented. Public

---

[4] Lewis spoke from her own experience and did not speak on behalf of the VA.

trust can be undermined by contradictory messaging and presentation of uncertain information as fact, she said.

When developing and framing communications, Krishnamurti said it can be very valuable to have a trusted source ask people about their experiences. This can help to expose logistical and psychosocial barriers to action that people might be facing (e.g., feeling stigmatized when attempting to dispose of medications at a police station). Interdisciplinary teams are also essential when developing communications and other behavioral interventions, she said. People with relevant experience should be included on teams from the start to help shape the questions to be asked and to identify needs.

Finally, and perhaps most importantly, Krishnamurti said that "any intervention or any communication has to be pretested, often iteratively, before there is any kind of wide scale roll-out." Testing need not be lengthy, complex, or expensive, she noted. Her research has shown how messages that experts think are obvious and clear might not be interpreted in the same way by non-experts (e.g., there are some perceptions that "FDA approved" means the agency recommends the product). She suggested that systematic pretesting of communications about REMS modifications should be required.

Motivating Disposal Behavior

A theme throughout the discussion of how to motivate people to dispose of unused opioids was the importance of making disposal easy. Brummett said studies and anecdotal reports suggest that "making something in-home and easy just seems to be the strongest and most important factor." Shamp concurred and noted the need to communicate to patients that disposal is easy. He added that making the process simple applies to motivating prescriber behavior as well. For example, there has been broad adoption of online registration for REMS prescriber certification versus the old method of filling out a paper form and faxing it. For online registration, prescribers enter their national provider identifier (NPI) and the webform is automatically populated with information from the NPI registry. Tsatoke agreed that ease of disposal is very important and said that disposal behavior in rural communities can be impacted by transportation-related issues. For the pilot study she discussed, having a community health representative visit patients at home and show them how to use the disposal bag made it very easy. She added that messaging about disposal should be tailored to the population (e.g., presented in Tribal languages with culturally appropriate graphics). Krishnamurti agreed and said the focus has been on the patient, but it is also important to consider the larger context, specifically opportunities for social support and how the role of a patient's support circle in motivating disposal might be made easier.

Lewis said that education is another key component in increasing motivation to dispose. This includes raising awareness about the potential for misuse and diversion of unused opioids and highlighting the community benefit aspect of safe disposal. She pointed out that there can be "more than just one lever" to increase motivation and highlighted the need for a toolkit of strategies to motivate disposal behaviors.

Near-Term Actions

Panelists discussed near-term actions that could make an impact now, while longer-term strategies are developed (i.e., not letting the perfect be the enemy of the good), and opportunities for evaluating interventions.

Nicholson reiterated the opinion of NACDS that the best short-term solution is having a variety of disposal options available to consumers and providing education about those options, particularly how and why to use them. He observed that uptake of some options is better than others and perhaps real-world testing of what solutions consumers prefer could be done. He referred to the Iowa program again as a model as it provided financial motivation not only for patients (free disposal systems) but also for pharmacies (reimbursement for disposal systems and patient education services).

Brummett said the RCTs he discussed showed about 60 percent uptake of a provided in-home disposal kit (somewhat higher in the pediatric study), which was a positive finding versus controls, but also shows there are opportunities for improvement. He proposed studying how best to "nudge people into higher compliance" and identifying the many touchpoints in the health system where information about opioid disposal could be imparted (e.g., following surgery). He said many programs are already in place in which opioid disposal options are being promoted or dispensed and that these could be leveraged for studies in the shorter term. He suggested that studies could be done by overlaying randomization with regard to type of intervention or behavioral nudge used to better understand what motivates uptake and use in the intended population (i.e., not in patients prescribed opioids for chronic pain management). Participants and panelists discussed that RCTs comparing uptake of mailback envelopes to other disposal options, including in-home disposal systems, would be informative for FDA.

Lewis agreed that there are many touchpoints in the course of patient care that could be leveraged to evaluate how a particular intervention might improve uptake of opioid disposal (e.g., does discussion of opioid disposal options during post discharge follow-up increase the likelihood of disposal?). She also highlighted the need to "be attentive to potential unintended outcomes" when implementing and evaluating an intervention. As an example, Lewis said the VA has implemented a requirement for a risk review when prescribing an opioid to an opioid-naïve patient for more than a 5-day supply of an opioid. "Knowing that they will have to do a risk review if they prescribe more than 5 days has vastly decreased the number of prescriptions that are more than 5 days," she said.

Krishnamurti said there are multiple touchpoints in the health care system following a procedure for which a patient is prescribed an opioid that present opportunities for communication about in-home disposal (e.g., interactions with prescribing physicians, pharmacists, physical therapists, home health aides conducting follow-up visits). "Some of those touchpoints are going to be more effective than others, but just pairing that behavior with something that is going to happen anyway is going to be a high-yield opportunity," she said. Discharge nurses are an example of a trusted follow-up touchpoint, observed Brummett. He suggested that providing a disposal system and associated education might be more readily protocolized as part of the work of the discharge nurse or the pharmacist dispensing the opioid, or possibly included in a postoperative phone call. Nicholson raised the issue of whether an ICD-10 code would be needed for protocolization of these services. Lewis said, "The VA has 139 different health care systems" and is a ready partner for research and evaluation on this issue.

Tsatoke reiterated that the community health representatives in Tribal communities are trusted touchpoints in the spectrum of health services. They conduct follow-up visits as well as many other health-related activities (e.g., helping to correctly install a car seat). This presents near-term opportunities to work with partners to implement pilot programs encouraging opioid disposal. For example, in-home disposal systems could be distributed through Tribal behavioral health programs that work with parents and caregivers of teens at high risk for misuse of opioids. Tsatoke encouraged participants to engage Tribal representatives as partners in these initiatives and in discussions of resources.

Nicholson said there are examples of pharmacies partnering with community organizations to implement a drug disposal kiosk in the pharmacy. Funding from states and from manufacturer product stewardship programs can also support pharmacies in providing patient education about opioid disposal. Nicholson also highlighted the need to engage health plans and payers as they could have a role in changing patient behavior by providing reimbursement to prescribers and dispensers for services related to educating patients about opioids.

Shamp pointed out that developing a REMS modification is generally not a simple task, and implementation and evaluation occurs over the longer term. Shamp also suggested partnering with payers as they have information on who has been prescribed opioids. As another near-term action, payers could text these patients at regular intervals to remind them of how they can dispose of any unused opioids from their prescription. As discussed, it can be very difficult for patients to find useful information about disposal, and this would be one way to make disposal easy.

Sharon Wrona, a pediatric nurse practitioner, said there is a need for educational materials that are targeted to families. She referred participants to a video about home opioid safety from Nationwide Children's Hospital that is shown on their inpatient video system and that they share nationally through the GetWellNetwork.

9

Reflections on the Design and Implementation of In-Home Opioid Disposal Systems

---

Highlights of Key Points Made by Individual Speakers*

- A multipronged approach is needed to remove unused opioids from the home. No one method will meet all needs. (Bix, Horwitz, Raulerson)
- Promoting a culture in which opioid disposal replaces opioid retention as the norm is a key element for the success of any drug disposal system. (Horwitz, Raulerson)
- Clear and consistent messaging is needed regarding the importance of safe opioid disposal, the in-home drug disposal systems available, and how to appropriately use them. (Coop, Raulerson)
- Disposal systems should be easy to use, effective, and safe for the user, household members, pets, and the environment. Minimum criteria for in-home disposal systems are needed and could include clarity of instructions and ease of use, non-toxic and non-hazardous components including final product–drug mixtures, ability to alter the physical integrity of the formulation such that the active pharmaceutical ingredient can be rendered unusable, and ability to deter misuse. (Coop, McGinty, Raulerson)
- It will be necessary to know the specific components of the disposal systems to evaluate the safety and effectiveness of in-home drug disposal systems. (McGinty, Wood)

- Studies are needed to understand the impact of concurrent disposal of both opioid and non-opioid medications on the safety and effectiveness of in-home disposal systems. (Coop, Wood)
- It is critical to engage trusted partners, such as physicians and pharmacists, in providing education and disposal solutions to patients. (Bicket)
- The perspectives of consumers should be considered in the design and implementation of disposal systems. (Bicket, Egan)
- State, local, Tribal, and other programs that have experience with opioid disposal programs can inform the development of federal programs. Partner where appropriate to avoid creating conflicting programs. (Bicket, Wood)
- Barriers to the uptake and use of in-home opioid disposal systems could include costs, complexity, confusion about options, and perceptions about disposal system use. (McGinty)
- More studies are needed that directly compare the uptake and effectiveness of in-home systems to other disposal options. (Bicket, McGinty)
- Concerns persist about potential contamination of water supplies stemming from disposal of opioids in the solid waste/landfill system. (Grossman)
- Requiring dispensing of in-home disposal systems under the risk evaluation and mitigation strategy might conflict with state and local solid waste regulations. (McGinty)

*This list is the rapporteurs' summary of points made by the individual speakers identified, and the statements have not been endorsed or verified by the National Academies of Sciences, Engineering, and Medicine. They are not intended to reflect a consensus among workshop participants.

Beth McGinty, chief of the Division of Health Policy and Economics and professor in the Department of Population Health Sciences at Weill Cornell Medicine, shared her perspective on some of the key discussions from the workshop.

- **Evidence supporting use.** The clinical trials discussed during the workshop suggest that providing an in-home disposal system increases the likelihood of disposal versus controls. McGinty noted, however, that this research is still in the early stages and more studies are needed that directly compare the uptake of in-home systems to other disposal options (e.g., mail-back envelopes).

- **Barriers to use.** Several potential barriers to the uptake and use of in-home opioid disposal systems were discussed, such as costs for consumers, complexity of instructions and difficulty of use, confusion about what is the "best" option to use, and public perceptions about the end product–drug mixtures (e.g., environmental impacts), McGinty said.
- **Disposal system evaluation.** To evaluate the safety and effectiveness of in-home drug disposal systems, it will be necessary to know the specific components of the systems, she continued. Disposal system testing will be complicated by the likelihood that patients will also dispose of non-opioid medications in these products.
- **Minimum criteria for disposal systems.** Should FDA decide to exercise its REMS authority to require dispensing of in-home drug disposal systems with prescribed opioids, minimum criteria for these systems will need to be determined, McGinty said. Several potential criteria were discussed, such as the extent to which a system renders opioids unusable; deters recovery of drug from the end product–drug mixture after disposal; and is safe for the user, household members, pets, and the environment.
- **Overlapping regulatory authorities.** The legal and regulatory landscape for in-home drug disposal systems was also discussed. McGinty recalled discussions of how requiring dispensing of in-home disposable systems might conflict with state and local solid waste regulations that would prohibit discarding the used disposal kits in the trash.

PARTICIPANT REFLECTIONS

To conclude the workshop, Laura Bix, Patrick Raulerson, Andrew Coop, Mark Bicket, and Jeff Horwitz shared their reflections on recurring themes from across the five panel sessions in an open discussion moderated by Alastair Wood.

Developing a Multipronged Approach

Throughout the workshop several speakers discussed that opioids have a role in pain management, Wood said. There are ongoing efforts to promote appropriate prescribing, but patients frequently have unused drug remaining after treatment. Workshop discussions covered a range of approaches for removing unused opioids from the home in a timely manner, with a focus on the role of in-home drug disposal systems.

A consistent message across the discussions was that a multipronged approach to removing unused opioids from the home is needed, Bix said. There is no one system that will meet all needs. Raulerson agreed there is no single best option. The RCT evidence discussed suggests that providing patients with a disposal option and associated education promotes disposal, but evidence about which disposal option is best suited to which patient is lacking and emphasizes the need for a multipronged approach, he said. Different patients might be better served by one option over another, depending on personal needs and preferences. Raulerson pondered whether the collection of these types of data could be included in the REMS to inform future REMS modifications on the dispensing of disposal options.

Horwitz agreed that a multifaceted approach is needed, including taking all opportunities across the pathway of care to provide disposal systems and education as appropriate. William Simpson of DisposeRx expressed support for all solutions that contribute to addressing the issue of opioids in the community. He also emphasized the importance of sustained efforts to educate and raise awareness about the risks of opioids. There are opportunities to engage patients during encounters with physicians, nurses, or pharmacists, as well as through EHR systems, pharmacy apps, and the types of messaging strategies discussed by Kathleen Egan, he said.

Throughout the workshop lessons from FDA's current REMS modification on providing mail-back envelopes were discussed. FDA has received comments raising concerns about the implementation of the opioid mail-back program, particularly about the potential for diversion by USPS employees or others.[1] However, Raulerson pointed out that mail-back for other types of medications has been used safely for some time. He added that the USPS has ensured FDA that the regulations and internal policies and practices in place that apply to current mail-back programs will also ensure the safety of the mail-back of opioids, and systems are in place for response should any issues arise. Kristen Aldred of Stericycle concurred that mail-back programs and take-back kiosks have been used successfully in some states for the collection of unused medication.

Engaging All Stakeholders

Discussions highlighted the need to engage trusted partners, such as physicians and pharmacists, in providing education and disposal solutions to patients, Bicket said, and to learn from other stakeholders, including state, Tribal, and other programs that have experience with opioid disposal programs. It was also stated, Bix said, that the perspectives of consumers

---

[1] See https://www.fda.gov/drugs/news-events-human-drugs/our-perspective-cders-efforts-expand-opioid-disposal-options (accessed November 18, 2023).

need to be considered in disposal system design (to understand resources, barriers, and motivations that might impact uptake and use).

The complexities and challenges of implementing REMS requirements were discussed, and points were made about partnering with entities already involved in opioid disposal to help ensure that new requirements do not conflict with or supplant their efforts or create confusion, Bicket said. Wood added that examples of initiatives by individual states, such as those discussed at the workshop, can inform the development of federal programs. Raulerson said the agency is cognizant of this and wants to hear more from stakeholders about what has and has not worked.

Milton Dallas of Rx Destroyer noted that he and other industry attendees have significant experience to share in packaging and disposal systems. He urged decision makers to engage manufacturers of drug disposal systems in discussions about development and implementation of these systems. Dallas also suggested looking to industry for new solutions for the destruction of opioids beyond incineration (e.g., chemical digestion, other thermal destruction methods).

Bix suggested that the Consumer Product Safety Commission also be engaged in discussions, and that the issue of child-resistant packaging be discussed. Horwitz noted that some in-home disposal systems do have appropriate child-resistant closures.

Properties of In-Home Drug Disposal Systems

Minimum Criteria

Discussions of the minimum criteria that opioid disposal systems should meet emphasized the need for systems that can be "safely, effectively, and easily" used, Raulerson said, noting that ease of use is essential because "they have to be used to work."

Some of the minimum criteria for in-home disposal systems discussed, as summarized by Coop, were clarity of instructions and ease of use; non-toxic and non-hazardous components and product–drug mixtures; ability to deter misuse; and ability to alter the physical integrity of the formulation so that the active pharmaceutical ingredient can be rendered unusable. Coop noted that clarity is needed on how non-hazardous and non-toxic would be defined and measured. Another point from the discussion was how to develop in-home opioid disposal systems that account for the fact that people will likely dispose of many different medications in the systems.

Simpson noted the challenges that overlapping regulatory authority over opioid disposal presents for manufacturers of in-home systems. He supported the establishment of minimum criteria and said that having a clear message on standards from regulatory agencies would support innovation and better solutions.

Scientific Considerations

Summarizing the panel discussion on scientific considerations, Coop said that drugs disposed via mail-back programs are incinerated, which removes any concern about product–drug mixtures. However, ingredients in in-home disposal systems can react differently, depending on what is added to them. As discussed, for example, calcium hypochlorite is an oxidizer that can alter pharmaceuticals but can also be extremely hazardous if combined with certain substances (e.g., releasing chlorine gas or generating potentially carcinogenic compounds). It was discussed that studies are needed to understand how these disposal systems perform when various non-opioid medications are added, but that it is not practical to test against all possible medications people might choose to put in the kits. Using activated charcoal to adsorb active pharmaceutical ingredients could be a safe option, but Coop noted that a tablet or similar formulation must first be broken down to release the active pharmaceutical ingredient to be adsorbed. While he said it is unlikely that those seeking drugs would attempt to extract a small amount of opioid from a large volume of activated charcoal, concerns were raised about drug leaching into the environment in landfills.

Evaluation of Safety, Efficacy, and Effectiveness

In implementing a REMS requirement for dispensing of in-home opioid disposal systems, FDA will need information about the safety, efficacy, and effectiveness of these systems. It was noted throughout the workshop that assessing safety will require knowing all the components of an in-home disposal system, Wood said. It will also be important to evaluate the safety of the product–drug mixture because it might be retained in the home for a period of time.

Another point discussed, Wood said, was that studies of safety and effectiveness in real-world use should compare in-home disposal systems to appropriate controls (e.g., other drug removal or return options and associated educational information). As noted above, the need to understand how safety and efficacy of in-home disposal systems are affected by the concurrent disposal of both opioid and non-opioid medications in the same disposal system was also discussed.

Egan stressed the need for caution when establishing whether a disposal intervention works. When evaluating why a program has not worked as anticipated, it is necessary to ask whether the intervention, the implementation, or the evaluation did not work, she said. For example, some participants said mail-back programs do not work while others discussed successful programs. Comments to FDA indicate that there is a public perception that diversion will occur, and she suggested that this perception could be targeted and modified to potentially enhance success of the mail-back program.

Bix reiterated the importance of understanding how people interface with information on packaging. In her work she has observed "extraneous information interfering with people's ability to find and use information that they need." The absence of information can also lead to user confusion. For example, products containing latex must be labeled as such, but she has observed practitioners spending critical minutes searching for latex labeling on latex-free products to be sure they have not missed it.

Implementation and Motivating Behavioral Change

The need for clear and consistent messaging about the importance of opioid disposal and the options available was reiterated throughout the workshop, Coop said. Lewis Grossman also pointed out the importance of clarity, suggesting that it needs to be clearer that mail-back envelopes are a disposal method. The phrase "mail back" could be misinterpreted by patients as returning the medication they paid for to the manufacturer, perhaps to be sold again, he said. In response, Egan said this emphasizes the points made throughout the workshop about the importance of engaging consumers in product and program development.

The importance of ensuring that patients understand how to use in-home disposal systems safely and correctly was also discussed, Wood said, including the need for culturally appropriate education and implementation.

Opinions varied regarding the ability of consumers to safely follow kit instructions. Horwitz asserted that most disposal systems are quite simple to use, while Coop and Wood reiterated the concerns that were expressed about people not using kits as intended, with potentially hazardous outcomes. Wood also pointed out that it might not always be clear to patients which of the drugs they might want to dispose of are opioids and which are not (just as patients often have difficulty identifying products that contain acetaminophen, which creates the potential for acetaminophen overdose). Horwitz emphasized the importance of bringing disposal options to the public to promote behavioral change and expressed faith that the American public will be able to safely follow the instructions. He likened disposal systems to other widely used consumer products that have educational campaigns to inform consumers of the risks if misused or not stored securely, such as laundry detergent pods.[2]

An element of all the disposal efforts discussed is the need to change the entrenched patient behavior of retaining unused prescribed opioids after treatment is no longer needed, Raulerson said. Various reasons why patients keep unused drugs were discussed, as well as strategies to nudge or push patients toward medication disposal. In this regard, the importance of education about the need for opioid disposal and how to dispose was emphasized throughout the workshop, Raulerson said, including the need for this information to be reinforced at as many touchpoints as possible (e.g., the practitioner/prescriber, the pharmacist/dispenser, automated text-based reminders, public health campaigns). Timely patient education is part of a multifaceted approach, and simply providing additional disposal options is not likely to significantly increase the prevalence of disposal, he said.

Horwitz agreed that promoting culture change around opioid disposal is a key element for the success of any disposal options. He said mail-back programs and kiosks "work to a point" in removing medications from homes, but they are not working in the broader sense that they are not motivating widespread behavioral change toward increased disposal of opioids.

Incentives that might motivate disposal behavior were discussed throughout the workshop. Studies suggest that financial incentives and convenience can be effective motivators to some extent. Although options such as mailing, dropping off, or flushing are all easy to do, people are still not motivated to do them, Horwitz said. In many cases, he added, disposal is unfortunately motivated by a personal opioid-related concern or loss (e.g., family member addiction or overdose).

Bicket said incentives to promote a particular clinician behavior or action in association with opioid prescribing must be carefully considered so that they do not inadvertently encourage increased opioid prescribing. He highlighted the many points made about the need for supportive materials and a team approach involving trusted practitioners along the patient's care pathway (e.g., educational materials for use at discharge prescribing).

Covering the Costs of In-Home Opioid Disposal

Simpson said that the costs of in-home disposal systems are currently paid by the customers—that is, those who distribute the systems (e.g.,

---

[2] See https://www.cpsc.gov/s3fs-public/390%20Laundry%20Packets.pdf (accessed November 18, 2023).

pharmacies, universities, health systems). He noted that these customers generally distribute the disposal systems for free, but there are instances in which the consumer is paying for the system. Horwitz added that there are coalitions using donor funding to purchase in-home disposal systems for distribution, and he has worked with businesses that purchase them for employees. Mary Kellington noted that the Washington state program she discussed is entirely funded by drug manufacturers.

Simpson said securing reimbursement from payers is a challenging process. In the absence of reimbursement, the costs of making in-home disposal systems available could be paid by the manufacturers of opioid analgesics; by pharmacy stewardship programs; out of opioid settlements; by government payers; by companies through their environmental, social, and corporate governance programs; or most likely, by a combination of sources. Simpson noted that manufacturer costs "trickle down to the patient eventually."

Raulerson suggested that if in-home disposal systems were to be required under the REMS, then the costs would be paid by the opioid manufacturers. He agreed with Simpson that costs are often shifted to the consumer but added that "disposal should be considered a fundamental safety attribute of the product" similar to the manufacturing processes that ensure the quality and stability of the drug. The manufacturer bears all costs of producing the product, which is ultimately reflected in the price.

Environmental Considerations

Grossman reviewed some of the environmental considerations raised throughout the workshop, including concerns about potential contamination of water supplies stemming from flushing and from disposal in the solid waste/landfill system. It was also discussed that EPA prefers incineration for the disposal for medications, he recalled. The challenge is how to balance these environmental concerns with the urgent need to increase the timely removal of unused opioids from circulation. Wood said the risk to the environment is likely to be significantly less than the risk of overdose associated with consumption of opioids in the home. Wood, Coop, and Kristin Fitzgerald all pointed out that opioids are also released into the wastewater system via excretion.

Raulerson acknowledged the need "to consider what patients and health care practitioners and pharmacists think about the ... differential environmental impacts of these various options." Contradictory guidance from FDA versus local governments (e.g., with regard to flushing) also needs to be considered when deciding how best to reduce exposure to opioids.

K. Fitzgerald added that EPA and FDA have discussed the messaging around flushing. "We recognize FDA has this flush list," she said, and there are select situations where flushing is applicable. The flush list is intended for homes with small children or pets to facilitate disposal of generally small quantities of drugs that are "potentially fatal in low doses," she said.

Topics for Further Research and Discussion

Bicket highlighted the need to direct funding toward filling the gaps in research discussed in the session on the role of in-home opioid disposal systems. Some of the areas highlighted included understanding what motivates or dissuades disposal behaviors (e.g., the studies discussed of messaging strategies), and comparative effectiveness studies of disposal options.

Bicket also summarized some of the other questions raised that need further attention, including the following: What are potential unintended consequences of requiring another disposal option under the REMS (e.g., creating confusion about which method to choose)? Who covers the costs of in-home disposal, and is there a role for payers? What other groups can support in-home disposal? What can be done from a harm reduction perspective to change the culture from one of retaining opioids to one where disposing is the norm? Another question, Raulerson said, is if multiple disposal options were included under the REMS, who drives the decision of which disposal option a patient receives? Should it be the patient, clinician, pharmacist, manufacturer, payer, and/or FDA?

References

Agarwal, A. K., Z. S. Ali, B. Sennett, R. Xiong, J. Hemmons, E. Spencer, H. Lacko, E. Hume, S. Mehta, and M. K. Delgado. 2021. An automated text messaging program to inform postoperative opioid prescribing. *New England Journal of Medicine Catalyst Innovations in Care Delivery* 2(3).

Agarwal, A. K., D. Lee, Z. Ali, Y. Wu, M. Coniglio, T. Uritsky, and M. K. Delgado. 2022. Effect of mailing an at-home disposal kit on unused opioid disposal after surgery: A randomized clinical trial. *Journal of the American Medical Association Network Open* 5(5):e2210724.

Bicket, M. C., J. J. Long, P. J. Pronovost, G. C. Alexander, and C. L. Wu. 2017. Prescription opioid analgesics commonly unused after surgery: A systematic review. *Journal of the American Medical Association Surgery* 152(11):1066-1071.

Bicket, M. C., D. Fu, M. D. Swarthout, E. White, S. A. Nesbit, and C. L. Monitto. 2021. Effect of drug disposal kits and fact sheets on elimination of leftover prescription opioids: The DISPOSE multi-arm randomized controlled trial. *Pain Medicine* 22(4):961-969.

Bix, L., N. M. Bello, R. Auras, J. Ranger, and M. K. Lapinski. 2009. Examining the conspicuousness and prominence of two required warnings on OTC pain relievers. *Proceedings of the National Academy of Sciences USA* 106(16):6550-6555.

Brummett, C. M., R. Steiger, M. Englesbe, C. Khalsa, J. J. DeBlanc, L. R. Denton, and J. Waljee. 2019. Effect of an activated charcoal bag on disposal of unused opioids after an outpatient surgical procedure: A randomized clinical trial. *Journal of the American Medical Association Surgery* 154(6):558-561.

Butler, C., Z. Kornberg, and H. L. Copp. 2021. Practitioner counseling associated with improved opioid disposal among families of postoperative pediatric patients. *Journal of Pediatric Urology* 17(5):634.e1-634.e7.

de la Fuente, J., and L. Bix. 2011. A tool for designing and evaluating packaging for healthcare products. *Journal for Patient Compliance* 1(1):48-52.

Draper, P., J. Bleicher, J. K. Kobayashi, E. L. Stauder, G. J. Stoddard, J. E. Johnson, J. N. Cohan, K. A. Kaphingst, A. H. S. Harris, and L. C. Huang. 2022. Patient willingness to dispose of leftover opioids after surgery: A mixed methods study. *Annals of Surgery Open* 3(4):e223.

Egan, K. L., M. Wolfson, K. M. Lukacena, C. M. Zelaya, M. S. McLeary, and D. W. Helme. 2020. Developing a health communication campaign for disposal of unused opioid medications. *Addictive Behaviors Reports* 12:100291.

Egan, K. L., C. A. Johnston, J. T. Jackson, S. E. Foster, and J. G. L. Lee. 2022. Rates and correlates of medicine disposal program implementation at pharmacies in North Carolina: A longitudinal study, 2016-2021. *Journal of the American Pharmacists Association* 62(4):1329-1337.

Gaw, C. E., A. E. Curry, K. C. Osterhoudt, J. N. Wood, and D. J. Corwin. 2023. Characteristics of fatal poisonings among infants and young children in the United States. *Pediatrics* 151(4):e2022059016.

Harbaugh, C. M., P. Malani, E. Solway, M. Kirch, D. Singer, M. J. Englesbe, C. M. Brummett, and J. F. Waljee. 2020. Self-reported disposal of leftover opioids among U.S. adults 50-80. *Regional Anesthesia & Pain Medicine* 45(12):949-954.

Helme, D. W., K. L. Egan, K. M. Lukacena, L. Roberson, C. M. Zelaya, M. S. McCleary, and M. Wolfson. 2020. Encouraging disposal of unused opioid analgesics in Appalachia. *Drugs: Education, Prevention and Policy* 27(5):407-415.

Hendricks, M. A., S. El Ibrahimi, G. A. Ritter, D. Flores, M. A. Fischer, R. D. Weiss, D. A. Wright, and S. G. Weiner. 2023. Association of household opioid availability with opioid overdose. *Journal of the American Medical Association Network Open* 6(3):e233385.

Huang, L. C., J. E. Johnson, J. Bleicher, A. N. Blumling, M. Savarise, D. W. Wetter, J. N. Cohan, A. A. S. Harris, and K. A. Kaphingst. 2023. Promoting disposal of left-over opioids after surgery in rural communities: A qualitative description study. *Health Education & Behavior* 50(2):281-289.

Lawrence, A. E., A. J. Carsel, K. L. Leonhart, H. W. Richards, C. M. Harbaugh, J. F. Waljee, D. J. McLeod, P. C. Walz, P. C. Minneci, K. J. Deans, and J. N. Cooper. 2019. Effect of drug disposal bag provision on proper disposal of unused opioids by families of pediatric surgical patients: A randomized clinical trial. *Journal of the American Medical Association Pediatrics* 173(8):e191695.

Lipari, R. N., and A. Hughes. 2017. How people obtain the prescription pain relievers they misuse. *The CBHSQ Report*. Center for Behavioral Health Statistics and Quality, Substance Abuse and Mental Health Services Administration.

Liu, L. 2016. The effect of labeling content and prominence on information processing among older adults during self-selection of over-the-counter medications. PhD Diss., Michigan State University.

Mallama, C. A., C. Greene, A. A. Alexandridis, J. K. McAninch, G. Dal Pan, and T. Meyer. 2022. Patient-reported opioid analgesic use after discharge from surgical procedures: A systematic review. *Pain Medicine* 23(1):29-44.

Otufowora, A., K. L. Egan, P. V. Chaudhari, A. A. Okusanya, A. O. Ogidan, and L. B. Cottler. 2023 (in press). Drug deactivation pouches for primary prevention of opioid overdose: Perceptions and attitudes of community members in North Central Florida. *Journal of the American Board of Family Medicine*.

Skaggs, C. S., and B. A. Logue. 2022. The prevalence of opioids in U.S. drinking water sources detected using direct-injection high-performance liquid chromatography-tandem mass spectrometry. *Environmental Toxicology and Chemistry* 41(11):2658-2666.

Tsatoke, A., R. Morones, I. Ampadu, and M. Stephens. 2021. Prescription drug safe storage practices in Arizona tribal communities. *Injury Prevention* 27(4):379-383.

West, B. A., R. A. Rudd, E. K. Sauber-Schatz, and M. F. Ballesteros. 2021. Unintentional injury deaths in children and youth, 2010-2019. *Journal of Safety Research* 78:322-330.

Appendix A

Workshop Agenda

DEFINING AND EVALUATING IN-HOME DISPOSAL SYSTEMS FOR OPIOID ANALGESICS

DAY 1: JUNE 26, 2023

9:00 a.m. **Welcome and Opening Remarks**
ALASTAIR WOOD, *Workshop Co-Chair*
Professor of Medicine Emeritus
Vanderbilt University School of Medicine

9:05 a.m. **FDA Authority for In-Home Opioid Disposal**
MARTA SOKOLOWSKA
Deputy Center Director for Substance Use and Behavioral Health
Center for Drug Evaluation and Research
Food and Drug Administration

9:15 a.m. **Fireside Chat: Life Cycle of Prescribed Opioids**
ROBERT HOFFMAN, *Speaker*
Professor, Department of Emergency Medicine
New York University Grossman School of Medicine

BETH McGINTY, *Workshop Co-Chair, Moderator*
Chief, Division of Health Policy and Economics
Professor, Department of Population Health Sciences
Weill Cornell Medicine

SESSION I — ENVISIONING DISPOSAL SYSTEMS TO REMOVE OPIOIDS FROM THE HOME

Session Objectives:

- Describe the properties or characteristics that an ideal in-home disposal system might possess such that it minimizes barriers to patient use.
- Consider under what circumstances people will use an in-home disposal system, with a focus on conditions that impede use and how those can be overcome.
- Discuss how human-centered design can inform the goals, development, and use of in-home disposal systems.
- Discuss health equity considerations in developing and implementing in-home disposal systems.

9:55 a.m. **Presentation**
LAURA BIX
Assistant Dean for Teaching, Learning and Academic Analytics
Michigan State University College of Agriculture & Natural Resources

10:15 a.m. **Panel Discussion**
RUCHI FITZGERALD, *Moderator*
Assistant Professor, Rush University
Service Chief of Inpatient Addiction Medicine, PCC Community Wellness Center

Panelists

Health Care Innovation Perspective
ANISH AGARWAL
Assistant Professor of Emergency Medicine
University of Pennsylvania Perelman School of Medicine

Behavioral Science Perspective
KATHLEEN EGAN
Assistant Professor, Health Education and Promotion
East Carolina University College of Health and Human
   Performance

Consumer/Patient Perspective
LINDSAY BARAN
Senior Research Director
Health Care Evaluation Department
NORC at the University of Chicago

Opioid Stewardship Perspective
LYEN HUANG
Assistant Professor of Surgery
University of Utah Spencer Fox Eccles School of Medicine

11:15 a.m.   **BREAK** (*30 mins*)

SESSION II — REGULATORY LANDSCAPE FOR HOUSEHOLD OPIOID DISPOSAL

Session Objectives:

- Examine the current landscape of laws and regulations that apply to in-home drug disposal systems.
- Explore the role of state and local policies on drug disposal and how FDA regulations may interact with those policies, including any unintended consequences.
- Consider the intersection of federal, state, and local waste disposal policies regarding the use of in-home disposal systems for opioid analgesics.

11:45 a.m.   **Presentation**
                HANZ ATIA
                Associate, Policy and Programs
                Product Stewardship Institute

12:05 p.m.   **Panel Discussion**
                LEWIS GROSSMAN, *Moderator*
                Professor
                American University Washington College of Law

Panelists

EPA Regulatory Perspective
KRISTIN FITZGERALD
Environmental Protection Specialist
Office of Resource Conservation and Recovery
Environmental Protection Agency

State Drug Disposal Policy Perspective
MARY KELLINGTON
Safe Medication Return Program Manager
Washington State Department of Health

FDA Regulatory Perspective
PATRICK RAULERSON
Senior Regulatory Counsel
Center for Drug Evaluation and Research
Food and Drug Administration

Former Federal Opioid Policy Perspective
UTTAM DHILLON
Partner
Michael Best & Friedrich LLP

1:05 p.m. **LUNCH BREAK** (*55 mins*)

SESSION III — SCIENTIFIC CONSIDERATIONS FOR IN-HOME OPIOID DISPOSAL

Session Objectives:

- Identify ideal characteristics of an in-home disposal system from a mechanistic, safety, and environmental perspective.
- Explore the scientific considerations for in-home drug disposal systems that could be used to remove unused opioid analgesics from the home.
- Discuss what is known/unknown about available and developing methods (e.g., sequestration, adsorption, absorption) by which in-home disposal systems work, assuming the product is used as intended.
- Discuss scientific approaches for assessing and gathering data on the environmental impact of in-home drug disposal systems.

2:00 p.m.	**Presentation** MARGARET SHIELD Owner and Principal Community Environmental Health Strategies LLC
2:20 p.m.	**Panel Discussion** JESSICA YOUNG, *Moderator* Chief, Recycling and Generator Branch Environmental Protection Agency

Panelists

Opioid Chemistry Perspective
ANDREW COOP
Professor, Pharmaceutical Sciences
Associate Dean for Academic Affairs
University of Maryland School of Pharmacy

Toxicology Perspective
KAITLYN BROWN
Clinical Managing Director
America's Poison Centers

FDA Perspective
MARTA SOKOLOWSKA
Deputy Center Director for Substance Use and Behavioral Health
Center for Drug Evaluation and Research
Food and Drug Administration

Environmental Chemistry Perspective
PAUL BRADLEY
Project Lead
Drinking-Water and Wastewater Infrastructure Integrated Science Team
Ecosystems Mission, Environmental Health Program
U.S. Geological Survey

3:20 p.m.	**BREAK** (*30 mins*)

SESSION IV — REAL-WORLD USE AND IMPLEMENTATION OF IN-HOME OPIOID DISPOSAL SYSTEMS

Session Objectives:

- Consider what approaches/methodologies are needed to evaluate the safe and correct use of in-home drug disposal systems in real-world settings.
- Explore approaches for engaging consumers on how to use in-home disposal systems safely and as intended.
- Consider best practices to promote safe and effective use of in-home disposal systems, including the roles of clinicians, prescribers, and pharmacists.
- Discuss use studies to lay out tangible examples of unintended consequences.

3:50 p.m. **Presentation**
CHAD BRUMMETT
Bert N. LaDu Professor of Anesthesiology
Co-Director, Opioid Research Institute
Co-Director, Opioid Prescribing Engagement Network
University of Michigan Medical School

4:10 p.m. **Panel Discussion**
MARK BICKET, *Moderator*
Assistant Professor
Director, Pain & Opioid Research
Department of Anesthesiology
Institute for Healthcare Policy and Innovation
University of Michigan Medical School

Panelists

Implementation Perspective
ANDREA TSATOKE
Injury Prevention Specialist
Indian Health Service, Headquarters

Program Evaluation Perspective
ELEANOR T. LEWIS
Deputy Director, Program Evaluation & Resource Center
U.S. Department of Veterans Affairs

REMS Design and Implementation Perspective
JAMES SHAMP
Vice President for Data Intelligence & Program Analytics
United BioSource LLC

Retail Pharmacy Perspective
KEVIN NICHOLSON
Vice President, Public Policy, Regulatory, and Legal Affairs
National Association of Chain Drug Stores

Behavioral Science and Communication Perspective
TAMAR KRISHNAMURTI
Assistant Professor, Medicine and Clinical and Translational Science
Department of Medicine Center for Research on Health Care
University of Pittsburgh

5:20 p.m. **Summary Remarks**
ALASTAIR WOOD, *Workshop Co-Chair*

5:30 p.m. **DAY 1 ADJOURN**

DAY 2: JUNE 27, 2023

8:30 a.m. **Welcome and Opening Remarks**
BETH McGINTY, *Workshop Co-Chair*

8:50 a.m. **Risk Evaluation and Mitigation Strategies: An Overview**
LYNN MEHLER
Practice Area Lead, Pharmaceuticals & Biotechnology
Hogan Lovells LLP

SESSION V — THE ROLE OF IN-HOME OPIOID DISPOSAL

Session Objectives:
- Consider the role of an ideal in-home disposal system in addressing the public health goal of mitigating the risk of non-medical use or overdose associated with opioids.
- Discuss how previous workshop discussions may inform the design, implementation, and evaluation of in-home disposal systems.

- Consider data needs and practical approaches for assessing the use and effectiveness of disposal systems in real-world settings.

9:15 a.m.   **Presentation**
KATHLEEN EGAN
Assistant Professor, Health Education and Promotion
East Carolina University College of Health and Human Performance

9:35 a.m.   **Panel Discussion**
ROBERT MORONES, *Moderator*
Injury Prevention Specialist
Indian Health Service (Phoenix Area)
U.S. Department of Health and Human Services

Panelists
Pediatric Injury Prevention Perspective
CHRISTOPHER GAW
Pediatric Emergency Medicine Fellow
Associate Fellow, Center for Injury Research and Prevention
Children's Hospital of Philadelphia

Overdose Prevention Perspective
JEFF HORWITZ
Chief Executive Officer
SAFE Project

Harm Reduction Perspective
SUSAN SHERMAN
Bloomberg Professor of American Health
Department of Health, Behavior and Society
Johns Hopkins Bloomberg School of Public Health

National Institute on Drug Abuse Perspective
WILSON COMPTON
Deputy Director, National Institute on Drug Abuse
National Institutes of Health

10:45 a.m.   **BREAK** (*30 mins*)

APPENDIX A

SYNTHESIS DISCUSSION

Purpose:

- Integrate information gathered throughout the workshop in a discussion on the properties and characteristics of an ideal in-home disposal system, factors impacting implementation, and regulatory considerations for household opioid disposal.

11:15 a.m.   **Moderated Panel Discussion**
ALASTAIR WOOD, *Workshop Co-Chair, Moderator*

Panelists

Pharmaceutical Sciences Perspective
ANDREW COOP
Professor, Pharmaceutical Sciences
Associate Dean for Academic Affairs
University of Maryland School of Pharmacy

Implementation Perspective
MARK BICKET
Assistant Professor
Director, Pain & Opioid Research
Department of Anesthesiology
Institute for Healthcare Policy and Innovation
University of Michigan Medical School

Overdose Prevention Perspective
JEFF HORWITZ
Chief Executive Officer
SAFE Project

Human-Centered Design Perspective
LAURA BIX
Assistant Dean for Teaching, Learning and Academic Analytics
Michigan State University College of Agriculture & Natural Resources

Food and Drug Administration Perspective
PATRICK RAULERSON
Senior Regulatory Counsel
Center for Drug Evaluation and Research
Food and Drug Administration

12:15 p.m.   **Panel Discussion with Audience Engagement**

12:45 p.m.   **Closing Remarks**
BETH McGINTY, *Workshop Co-Chair*

1:00 p.m.   **DAY 2 ADJOURN**

Appendix B

Biographical Sketches of the Workshop Planning Committee Members, Speakers, and Panelists

PLANNING COMMITTEE BIOSKETCHES

Elizabeth McGinty, M.S., Ph.D. (*Co-Chair*), is the chief of the Division of Health Policy and Economics in the Department of Population Health Sciences at Weill Cornell Medicine. Dr. McGinty conducts health policy research related to mental health, substance use, and chronic pain and is a leading expert in prescription opioid policy. She has served on multiple prominent advisory groups, including a United Nations technical consultation panel on stigma reduction and drug use and a White House task force on suicide prevention. Dr. McGinty received her Ph.D. in health and public policy from the Johns Hopkins Bloomberg School of Public Health.

Alastair J. J. Wood, M.B., Ch.B., FRCP, FACP (*Co-Chair*), was professor of both medicine and pharmacology at Vanderbilt University School of Medicine and served as assistant vice chancellor for clinical research and associate dean before being appointed emeritus professor of medicine and emeritus professor of pharmacology. He served as the drug therapy section editor of the *New England Journal of Medicine* from 1985 to 2004. He was a partner at Symphony Capital LLC, a private equity company investing in the clinical development of novel biopharmaceutical products from 2006 to 2018 and was a member of the board of directors of the Critical Path Institute until 2022.

Dr. Wood has been honored by being elected to the National Academy of Medicine (formerly the Institute of Medicine); the American Association of Physicians; the American Society for Clinical Investigation; Honorary

Fellow, American Gynecological and Obstetrical Society; fellowship of the American College of Physicians; fellowship of the Royal College of Physicians of London; and fellowship of the Royal College of Physicians of Edinburgh. He was the 2005 recipient of the Rawls-Palmer Award and in 2008 received the honorary degree of Doctor of Laws, honoris causa, from the University of Dundee.

Dr. Wood is a past member of the Food and Drug Administration's Cardio-Renal Advisory Committee and the Non-Prescription Drug Advisory Committee, which he also chaired. He is currently an advisor to the Tufts University spin-off Immediate Therapeutics. Dr. Wood has served on a number of editorial boards and his research has resulted in more than 300 articles, reviews, and editorials.

Mark C. Bicket, M.D., Ph.D., FASA, is an assistant professor and director pain and opioid research in the Department of Anesthesiology and the Institute for Healthcare Policy and Innovation at the University of Michigan Medical School. He is also the co-director of the Opioid Prescribing Engagement Network, whose mission is to change the trajectory of the opioid crisis. Dr. Bicket and his colleagues have published around 100 peer-reviewed articles on prescription opioid use, non-opioid treatments for acute and chronic pain, the quality and safety of pain treatment in diverse health care settings, and clinical trials and health services research. He previously served on the National Academies of Sciences, Engineering, and Medicine Committee on Evidence-Based Clinical Practice Guidelines for Prescribing Opioids for Acute Pain. Dr. Bicket has provided scientific guidance on health care, opioid, and pain policy to government departments and agencies at the federal, regional, and state levels, including the White House Office of Science and Technology Policy and the Centers for Medicare & Medicaid Services. He previously directed the Fellowship Program and Quality and Safety for Pain Medicine at Johns Hopkins University (JHU), where he trained and mentored fellows, residents, and medical students while treating patients in East Baltimore. He received his M.D. and Ph.D. from JHU. He completed his anesthesiology residency at Johns Hopkins Hospital, where he served as chief resident, and his pain medicine fellowship training at Massachusetts General Hospital.

Irene Z. Chan, Pharm.D., is the deputy director in the Office of Medication Error Prevention and Risk Management within the Center for Drug Evaluation and Research (CDER) at the Food and Drug Administration (FDA). Previously, Captain (CAPT) Chan served as the director in the Division of Medication Error Prevention and Analysis I in CDER. CAPT Chan has expertise in regulatory science, human factors, risk management, and pharmacovigilance. CAPT Chan is responsible for managing, planning, and providing guidance for the premarket and postmarket operations, programs, functions, and activities of four Divisions in FDA that focus on minimizing use errors related to the naming, labeling, packaging, or design of drug products, and developing effective and efficient risk evaluation and mitigation strategies for certain drug products that ensure the benefits outweigh risks. She is also CDER's representative on the Association for the Advancement of Medical Instrumentation Human Factors Committee. CAPT Chan received B.S. in pharmacy and Doctor of Pharmacy degrees from Rutgers University Ernest Mario School of Pharmacy.

Ruchi M. Fitzgerald, M.D., FAAFP, is assistant professor in the Departments of Family Medicine and Psychiatry/Behavioral Sciences at Rush University. She is also the associate program director of the Rush University Addiction Medicine Fellowship. She is the service chief of Inpatient Addiction Medicine at PCC Community Wellness Center, a Federally Qualified Health Center system that serves the West Side of Chicago. Dr. Fitzgerald is a National Academy of Medicine James C. Puffer/American Board of Family Medicine fellow.

Dr. Fitzgerald's work has focused on promoting cross-sector collaboration to improve care for persons affected by substance use disorders, with an emphasis in the perinatal/child health arena. Her scholarly work has focused on addressing stigma, building capacity in primary care for treating opioid use disorder in special populations, and implementing evidence-based substance use disorder curricula in the next generation of clinicians.

Dr. Fitzgerald received her M.D. from the University of Michigan Medical School and completed her family medicine training with the Montana Family Medicine Residency and her Addiction Medicine Fellowship with Rush University.

Lewis Grossman, Ph.D., J.D., is the Ann Loeb Bronfman Professor of Law at the American University (AU) Washington College of Law, where he has taught since 1997 and where he served as associate dean for scholarship from 2008 to 2011. He teaches and writes in the areas of food and drug law, health law, American legal history, and civil procedure. He has also been a visiting professor of law at Cornell Law School and a Law and Public Affairs Fellow at Princeton University. Prior to joining the AU faculty, he was an associate at Covington & Burling LLP in Washington, DC. Before that, he clerked for Chief Judge Abner Mikva of the U.S. Court of Appeals for the DC Circuit. Professor Grossman's scholarship has appeared in the *Cornell Law Review*; *Law and History Review*; *Yale Journal of Health Policy, Law, & Ethics*; and *Administrative Law Review*, among others.

He has made recent contributions to volumes published by Oxford University Press and Columbia University Press. He is the co-author of *Food and Drug Law: Cases and Materials* (with Peter Barton Hutt and Richard A. Merrill) and of a widely used supplement to the first year civil procedure course titled *A Documentary Companion to A Civil Action* (with Robert G. Vaughn). In 2021, Oxford University Press will publish Professor Grossman's book titled *Choose Your Medicine: Freedom of Therapeutic Choice in America*. He has served as a member or legal consultant on three previous committees of the Health and Medicine Division (formerly the Institute of Medicine) of the National Academies of Sciences, Engineering, and Medicine. Professor Grossman earned his Ph.D. in history from Yale University, where he was awarded the George Washington Egleston Prize for Best Dissertation in the Field of American History. He received a J.D. magna cum laude from Harvard Law School and a B.A. summa cum laude from Yale University.

Stephen W. Hoag, Ph.D., is professor at the University of Maryland, Baltimore School of Pharmacy. He received a B.S. in biochemistry from the University of Wisconsin–Madison and a Ph.D. in pharmaceutical science from the University of Minnesota, Twin Cities. His primary research interests are in oral delivery systems, controlled release polymers, excipient functionality, stability testing, excipient functionality testing, abuse-deterrent formulations, pediatric formulations, and the use of Raman and near-infrared spectroscopy in process analytical technology applications. Dr. Hoag is the director of the School of Pharmacy Good Manufacturing Practices Facility, a member of the National Institute for Pharmaceutical Technology and Education Steering Committee for the Handbook of Pharmaceutical Excipients, a member of the editorial board of the journal called *Pharmaceutical Development and Technology*, and an American Association of Pharmaceutical Scientists Fellow.

Robert Morones, M.P.H., is the area injury prevention specialist for the Phoenix Area Indian Health Service (IHS). He is responsible for managing the Phoenix Area Injury Prevention Program, assisting more than 40 Arizona, California, Nevada, and Utah tribes and IHS professional staff in the development of community-based injury prevention programs and initiatives. Morones's past positions include being assigned as a service unit environmental health officer at the Fort Yuma Service Unit in Winterhaven, California, and as an environmental health specialist at the Centers for Disease Control and Prevention in Atlanta, GA. His educational background includes a B.S. in environmental health sciences from Wright State University and an M.P.H. from the University of Massachusetts at Amherst.

Thomas Prisinzano, Ph.D., received his B.S. in chemistry from the University of Delaware and his doctorate in pharmaceutical sciences from Virginia Commonwealth University. From 2000 to 2003, he was an Intramural Training Award Fellow in the National Institute of Diabetes and Digestive and Kidney Diseases. In 2003, Dr. Prisinzano began his career in the Division of Medicinal & Natural Products Chemistry in the College of Pharmacy at the University of Iowa. From 2007 to 2019, he was a faculty member in the Department of Medicinal Chemistry in the School of Pharmacy at the University of Kansas. In 2019, he joined the University of Kentucky College of Pharmacy. He currently serves as director of the Center for Pharmaceutical Research and Innovation and chair of the Pharmaceutical Sciences Department. His research combines medicinal and natural products chemistry. It is directed toward elucidation of the structure and function of neurotransmitter systems in the central nervous system in normal, drug-altered, and pathological states, and the development of medications for the treatment of drug abuse and pain.

Jessica Young, M.S., is the chief of the Recycling and Generator Branch in the Environmental Protection Agency's (EPA's) Office of Resource Conservation and Recovery within the Office of Land and Emergency Management. During her 17 years at EPA, Young has worked to ensure solid and hazardous waste are properly managed, recycled, and disposed. She has been the branch chief for 9 years. Her branch covers the cradle part of the Resource Conservation and Recovery Act cradle-to-grave hazardous waste regulations, including pharmaceutical waste issues, definition of solid waste recycling exclusions, hazardous waste generators, and more. She has earned EPA bronze awards for her work and leadership, including on the Hazardous Waste Pharmaceuticals Rule for Healthcare Facilities. Young earned a master's degree in environmental science and policy from John Hopkins University and a bachelor's degree in science of earth systems from Cornell University.

Patricia J. Zettler, J.D., is associate professor at The Ohio State University Moritz College of Law and a member of Ohio State's Drug Enforcement and Policy Center and its Comprehensive Cancer Center. Her research and teaching focus on Food and Drug Administration (FDA) law and policy, torts, and legislation and regulation. Her scholarship has appeared in leading legal and health sciences journals such as the *New England Journal of Medicine*, *Journal of the American Medical Association*, and *Science*, and has covered various topics, including expanded access, biohacking, stem cell interventions, opioids, cannabis products, tobacco and nicotine products, and COVID-19 countermeasures. Zettler also is a coauthor of the fifth edition of *Food and Drug Law: Cases and Materials* (with

Peter Barton Hutt, the late Richard A. Merrill, Lewis A. Grossman, Nathan Cortez, and Erika Lietzan). She currently serves on the Food and Drug Law Institute's Board of Directors and as co-chair of the International Society of Cell & Gene Therapy's Committee on the Ethics of Cell and Gene Therapy, also chairing its subcommittee on expanded access. Previously she served on the National Academies of Sciences, Engineering, and Medicine's (the National Academies') Committee on Reviewing the Public Health Emergency Medical Countermeasures Enterprise and as a consultant to the National Academies' Committee on Pain Management and Regulatory Strategies to Address Prescription Opioid Abuse. Before entering academics, Zettler served as an associate chief counsel in the Office of the Chief Counsel at FDA. She received her undergraduate and law degrees from Stanford University, both with distinction.

SPEAKER AND PANELIST BIOSKETCHES

Anish K. Agarwal, M.D., M.P.H., M.S., is assistant professor and chief wellness officer of emergency medicine at the University of Pennsylvania. His research interests fall at the intersection of health care delivery, innovation, and digital health. Dr. Agarwal seeks to use advancements in mobile health to help create and build learning health systems. His work specifically has been applied to the opioid epidemic, health care workforce well-being, and remote patient engagement.

Dr. Agarwal's work has been published in the *New England Journal of Medicine, Journal of the American Medical Association, Annals of Emergency Medicine, Journal of General Internal Medicine, Circulation, Resuscitation*, and *Critical Care Medicine*. His work has been featured throughout multiple media outlets. His work has been funded by the Food and Drug Administration, Agency for Healthcare Research and Quality, Patient-Centered Outcomes Research Institute, National Institutes of Health, and foundation grants. Dr. Agarwal completed his medical and public health training at the Tufts University School of Medicine and Public Health, followed by an emergency medicine residency at the University of Pennsylvania.

Hanz Atia, M.P.H., is an associate of policy and programs at the Product Stewardship Institute (PSI), a policy advocate and consulting non-profit that pioneered product stewardship in the United States. Atia completed an M.P.H. with a concentration in epidemiology and biostatistics from Tufts University, where they discovered how product stewardship blended their passion for public health and the environment. They joined PSI in 2022 to work on several product categories and now manage programs to expand take-back infrastructure for medical sharps and pharmaceuticals in Oklahoma and Missouri.

Lindsay Baran, M.S., is senior research director in the Health Care Evaluation department at NORC at the University of Chicago, where her work focuses on disability and health equity. Baran's background is in disability policy, and she has extensive experience in chronic pain and opioids policy and advocacy. Prior to her work at NORC, Baran worked as the policy director at the National Council on Independent Living, a national grassroots disability rights organization in Washington, DC, where she started the Chronic Pain and Opioids Task Force. She oversaw and implemented the organization's national policy and advocacy agenda. She currently serves as a board member for the National Pain Advocacy Center. Baran has lived with chronic pain for most of her life.

Baran currently works with the Centers for Medicare & Medicaid Services Office of Minority Health on several activities to improve health equity and reduce disparities. She also manages an evaluation of the Minnesota Department of Human Services' Home and Community–Based Services assessment process for racial and ethnic disparities. In addition, she manages a federal project to enhance data analysis and evidence-building capacity.

Earlier in her career, Baran worked at the National Center on Health Promotion Research for Persons with Disabilities, where she managed a study on the impact of improving the accessibility of health-related facilities and the built environment for people with disabilities.

Laura Bix, Ph.D., is assistant dean for teaching, learning, and academic analytics at Michigan State University College of Agriculture & Natural Resources and a professor at the School of Packaging at Michigan State University, where she leads the Packaging HUB (Healthcare, Universal Design, and Biomechanics). HUB researchers quantify the interface between people and packaging, with the goal of improving health outcomes by influencing both product design and policy. Her efforts have been recognized by an Excellence in Teaching Award, a Phi Kappa Phi Excellence in Interdisciplinary Scholarship Award, and appointment as an Academic Fellow to the Committee on Institutional Cooperation Academic Leadership Program. She has been an appointed expert to national and international panels convened by the International Organization for Standardization, the Food and Drug Administration, the Centers for Disease Control and Prevention, the Consumer Healthcare Products Association, and the Gerontological Society of America. She has also received distinction from industry as one of the 100 most notable people in the medical device industry named in *Medical Device and Diagnostics Magazine* in 2008. Dr. Bix completed her graduate education at Michigan State University.

Paul Bradley, Ph.D., M.S., is a research hydrologist with the U.S. Geological Survey (USGS), Ecosystems Mission, Environmental Health Program.

He is co-lead of the USGS Environmental Health Program, Drinking-Water and Wastewater Infrastructure Integrated Science Team. His research focuses on human exposures to and potential effects of inorganic, organic, and microbial contaminant mixtures in drinking water at the point of use and on exposures and adverse ecological health effects of stormwater and wastewater contaminant mixtures, including pharmaceuticals, on aquatic ecosystems. Dr. Bradley completed his master's in applied biology at the Georgia Institute of Technology and his doctorate in physiological ecology at the University of South Carolina.

Kaitlyn Brown, Pharm.D., DABAT, is the clinical managing director for America's Poison Centers. In this role, she promotes the use of poison center data by public health, industry, and non-government agencies to reduce poisoning. She serves on national committees that provide support for surveilling and responding to emerging hazards. As an adjunct assistant professor for the University of Utah and through her previous experience at the Utah Poison Control Center, she has contributed to clinical toxicology research and education. Dr. Brown holds a Doctor of Pharmacy degree from Wilkes University and completed a fellowship in clinical and applied toxicology at the Utah Poison Control Center. She is a Diplomate of the American Board of Applied Toxicology.

Chad M. Brummett, M.D., is professor at the University of Michigan Medical School where he serves as co-director of the Opioid Research Institute and as the senior associate chair for research. He has written or contributed to more than 270 publications, including articles in top journals such as *Journal of the American Medical Association* (JAMA), *JAMA Surgery*, *Anesthesiology*, and *Annals of Surgery*. He is also the co-director of the Opioid Prescribing Engagement Network (OPEN) at the University of Michigan, which aims to apply a preventative approach to the U.S. opioid epidemic through appropriate prescribing after surgery, dentistry, and emergency medicine, including opioid disposal. In addition, his research interests include predictors of acute and chronic postsurgical pain and failure to derive benefit from interventions and surgeries primarily to treat pain. He is the co-principal investigator of multiple National Institutes of Health grants studying these concepts. Dr. Brummett also receives funding from the Michigan Department of Health and Human Services, Substance Abuse and Mental Health Services Administration, Centers for Disease Control and Prevention, and multiple foundations. He completed his medical training at the Indiana University School of Medicine, a residency in anesthesiology at the University of Michigan Health System, and a fellowship in pain medicine at the Johns Hopkins Hospital.

Wilson Compton, M.D., M.P.E., is deputy director of the National Institute on Drug Abuse (NIDA) of the National Institutes of Health, where he has worked since 2002. Dr. Compton received his undergraduate education at Amherst College and medical education, including psychiatry training, at Washington University in St. Louis. Over his career, Dr. Compton has authored more than 250 publications and often speaks at high-impact venues. He was a member of DSM-5's Revision Task Force and has led, for NIDA, development of the Population Assessment of Tobacco and Health Study, jointly sponsored by NIDA and the Food and Drug Administration (FDA), with 45,971 participants. Dr. Compton has received multiple awards, including FDA awards for collaboration in 2012, 2013, and 2017, and the Health and Human Services Secretary's Awards for Meritorious Service in 2013 and Distinguished Service in 2015, 2018, and 2019.

Andrew Coop, Ph.D., is professor and associate dean for academic affairs at the University of Maryland School of Pharmacy. Dr. Coop has received funding from the National Institute on Drug Abuse for his chemistry research on opioids, stimulants, and depressants. Dr. Coop is a recipient of the Joseph Cochin Young Investigator Award from the College on Problems of Drug Dependence (CPDD) and is a Fellow of both the CPDD and the American Association of Pharmaceutical Scientists.

Dr. Coop served as the biological coordinator of the Drug Evaluation Committee of CPDD, where he coordinated with the Food and Drug Administration, Drug Enforcement Administration, and National Institute on Drug Abuse on obtaining biological data on compounds under emergency schedule to aid in final scheduling decisions.

He is sought for lectures on his expertise on the chemistry of opioids; has served as an expert witness in criminal trials; and testified before the U.S Senate Health, Education, Labor, and Pensions Committee on approaches to treat pain during the opioid crisis. Dr. Coop completed his doctorate in chemistry at the University of Bristol in England.

Uttam Dhillon, M.A., J.D., is an accomplished attorney with more than 30 years of legal experience, including more than 20 years in key roles within the federal government. Dhillon has served in high-profile positions at the White House, the Drug Enforcement Administration, the Department of Homeland Security, INTERPOL Washington, and the House of Representatives.

His law practice is centered on legislative and regulatory oversight, government investigations, and white-collar defense. In addition to his role as a partner at Michael Best, Dhillon is also a principal at Michael Best Consulting LLC. Previously, he was a co-founder and principal of DC Consulting LLC, a consulting firm specializing in law enforcement and drug-related issues. He completed his legal training at the University of California, Berkley School of Law.

Kathleen Egan, Ph.D., M.S., is assistant professor in the Department of Health Education and Promotion at East Carolina University. She completed a postdoctoral fellowship at the University of Florida Substance Abuse Training Center. She earned her Ph.D. in community health education from University of North Carolina at Greensboro and her M.S. in clinical and translational population science from Wake Forest University School of Medicine. Her overarching research agenda aims to reduce harms associated with substance use through the implementation of interventions and policies in medical, community, and academic settings. She has been funded by the National Institute on Drug Abuse (NIDA), Centers for Disease Control and Prevention (CDC), and Substance Abuse and Mental Health Services Administration to lead projects pertaining to secure storage and disposal of unused opioid medications.

Dr. Egan's research is focused on preventing harms associated with opioid, cannabis, and polysubstance use among adolescents and young adults. Her research involves the development and assessment of substance use prevention strategies that are implemented in community, medical, and academic settings. Dr. Egan is currently the principal investigator on a National Institutes of Health–funded R34 (NIDA) research study that aims to develop and pilot test a text message intervention to facilitate secure storage and disposal of unused prescription opioids (1R34DA051710-01). Her work is also supported by CDC and the North Carolina Division of Health and Human Services. Dr. Egan teaches program evaluation at both the undergraduate and graduate levels.

Kristin Fitzgerald, M.S., has been with the Environmental Protection Agency since 2001, working primarily on sector-based rule makings for hazardous waste generators. Fitzgerald started working with the Resource Conservation and Recovery Act (RCRA) more than 30 years ago, answering questions on the RCRA/Superfund Hotline. She holds a B.A. in government from St. Lawrence University and an M.S. in environmental science and policy from George Mason University.

Christopher Gaw, M.D., M.P.H., M.B.E., is a pediatric emergency medicine fellow and an associate fellow at the Center for Injury Research and Prevention at Children's Hospital of Philadelphia. Dr. Gaw's research is primarily on the epidemiology and prevention of pediatric injury and poisoning. In the past decade, he has worked with several research groups to study a wide array of topics, including head traumas, unintentional poisonings, and consumer product-related injuries. Dr. Gaw has significant experience leveraging large administrative databases to better characterize injury and poisoning hazards to children, with the goal of informing education, advocacy, and policy initiatives. His research also has used survey science and qualitative methods to understand provider views toward injury control. In addition to his injury prevention research, Dr. Gaw has academic interests in bioethics and medical education and has authored works on medical trainee wellness, shared decision making, and end-of-life care. He completed his doctoral training at the University of Pennsylvania Perelman School of Medicine, with a residency and fellowship at the Children's Hospital of Philadelphia.

Robert Hoffman, M.D., completed a 3-year internship and residency in internal medicine followed by a fellowship in medical toxicology, all at New York University (NYU) School of Medicine. He achieved and maintains Board Certification in Internal Medicine, Medical Toxicology, and Emergency Medicine. In 1989 Dr. Hoffman became director of the Fellowship in Medical Toxicology at the New York City Poison Center, and in 1994 he became director of the New York City Poison Center. He was director of the Division of Medical Toxicology at NYU School of Medicine from 2014 through 2020. Dr. Hoffman has authored more than 500 publications in peer-reviewed journals covering various aspects of toxicology. He has been an editor of *Goldfrank's Toxicologic Emergencies* for the past seven editions. Dr. Hoffman has held offices in all three American Toxicology Societies and is a recipient of the American College of Medical Toxicology Ellenhorn Award, the European Association of Poison Centres and Clinical Toxicologists Louis Roche Award, and the American Academy of Clinical Toxicology Career Achievement award. Dr. Hoffman's current interests focus on the development and propagation of evidence-based recommendations in toxicology. He is a co-chair of the Extracorporeal Treatments in Poisoning (EXTRIP) workgroup and the co-chair of the International Clinical Toxicology Recommendations Collaborative. In December 2022 Dr. Hoffman became the co-editor-in-chief of *Clinical Toxicology*. He completed his medical training at New York University.

Jeff Horwitz, J.D., M.S., joined SAFE Project in 2018 as the chief executive officer. He has 30 years of administrative, management, and leadership experience. SAFE Project is a national 501(c)(3) non-profit committed to overcoming the addiction epidemic in the United States. Founded by Admiral James and Mary Winnefeld in 2017 following the loss of their 19-year-old son Jonathan to an opioid overdose, SAFE Project provides transformative programming, training, and technical assistance based on a collaborative, multipronged, and nonpartisan approach within each of its key initiatives—SAFE Campuses, SAFE Communities, SAFE Workplaces, and SAFE Veterans.

Prior to arriving at SAFE Project, Horwitz served for 28 years in the U.S. Navy. He retired as a captain in 2014. In addition to his final assignment as the general counsel of the White House Military Office, Horwitz served in multiple assignments, including command judge advocate on board the USS Harry S. Truman (CVN 75); staff judge advocate, COMNAVAIRFOR; counsel for the commander, U.S. Naval Forces in Northern Europe and the United Kingdom; and director of the Navy's Legislative Program for nearly 9 years. In his free time, Horwitz serves on the board of St. Joseph's University's Center for Addiction and Recovery Education (CARE) and Heartshine, a resilience and trauma support community program in Harrisburg, PA. Horwitz earned a J.D. from the University of Pittsburgh, an M.S. in homeland security from American Military University, and a B.S. in international affairs from Seton Hall University.

Lyen Huang, M.D., M.P.H., FACS, FASCRS, is assistant professor of surgery at the Spencer Fox Eccles School of Medicine and adjunct assistant professor of family and preventative medicine and population health sciences at the University of Utah. He is a board-certified general and colorectal surgeon and provides care to patients with colorectal cancer, inflammatory bowel disease, and other gastrointestinal tract diseases. His research spans the breadth of perioperative opioid stewardship, including patient education, screening, patient-centered prescribing, prescribing guided by machine learning, transitional pain services, naloxone co-prescribing, and opioid disposal. He was a University of Utah Clinical and Translational Science Institute K12 Mentored Career Development Scholar from 2020 to 2022. Dr. Huang completed his medical training at Stanford University.

Mary Kellington joined the Washington State Department of Health in 2000 and began managing Washington's Safe Medication Return system in 2021. The impact of the environment on populations and of populations on the environment has intrigued Kellington throughout her public health career and informed her work developing and implementing public health programs. Her earlier work focused on maternal and infant health, adolescent health, and sexual and reproductive health. She enjoys working with a variety of stakeholders and facilitating collaboration among groups with conflicting priorities. She strives to make healthy choices easy choices.

Tamar Krishnamurti, Ph.D., is assistant professor of medicine at the University of Pittsburgh. Dr. Krishnamurti works on issues at the intersection of health, risk, technology, and communication. Dr. Krishnamurti was the 2020 recipient of the Kuno Award for Applied Science to develop mobile health strategies to address maternal morbidity and mortality risks. She leads the FemTech Collaborative at the University of Pittsburgh and is a cofounder of Naima Health, whose flagship product, MyHealthyPregnancy, offers early risk assessment and intervention for adverse pregnancy outcomes. Dr. Krishnamurti earned her Ph.D. in behavioral decision research at Carnegie Mellon University.

Eleanor T. Lewis, Ph.D., is deputy director of the Program Evaluation and Resource Center (PERC) in the Office of Mental Health and Suicide Prevention in the Veterans Administration (VA). PERC's mission is to use program evaluation and advanced informatics to promote more veteran-centered, effective, and cost-efficient care for veterans with mental health conditions and substance use disorders. In addition to supporting PERC's operational mission broadly, Dr. Lewis has participated in multiple research projects on opioid use and misuse and helped implement opioid safety and risk mitigation initiatives in the Department of Veterans Affairs for more than a decade. She helps lead implementation of the VA Stratification Tool for Opioid Risk Mitigation (STORM), which shows promise for targeting prevention interventions to reduce mortality in patients who are prescribed opioids. STORM was profiled on the Agency for Healthcare Research and Quality Patient Safety Network. Dr. Lewis earned her Ph.D. in organization science and sociology at Carnegie Mellon University.

Lynn Mehler, J.D., is a partner at Hogan Lovells LLP. As practice area lead for pharmaceuticals and biotechnology, Mehler advises clients on a range of Food and Drug Administration (FDA) and Drug Enforcement Administration (DEA) regulatory matters. She has worked extensively on the approval processes for new drugs and biologics, on safety issues that include risk evaluation and mitigation strategy (REMS), and on unique regulatory issues raised during the development and marketing of controlled substances. Drawing on her 12 years with the FDA's Office of the Chief Counsel, Mehler has a deep understanding of FDA. Her experience as the primary attorney handling all FDA issues related to controlled substances provides her with unique insights into both the FDA's and DEA's regulatory processes for controlled substances. She advised the agency on drug safety matters, including at approval and those leading to labeling changes, REMS, and even product withdrawal, and she applies that understanding to help clients create effective solutions for FDA regulatory matters.

Kevin Nicholson, R.Ph., J.D., is vice president of public policy, regulatory, and legal affairs for the National Association of Chain Drug Stores. In this role, he is responsible for the strategic direction of the association's public policy and regulatory affairs activities. Nicholson oversees activities and staff in providing legislative and regulatory policy analysis in federal and state health care issues. He and his team provide expertise to lobbyists and other association staff as well as chain members. He has more than 30 years of experience in the pharmacy industry, including 6 years as a practicing community pharmacist. Nicholson earned his J.D. at Tulane University Law School.

Patrick Raulerson, J.D., has been with the Food and Drug Administration (FDA) for 14 years, focusing on regulation of opioids, biosimilars, combination products, and medical gases. He has been part of FDA's efforts to work with Congress on several major pieces of legislation, including the SUPPORT Act, the 21st Century Cures Act, and Food and Drug Administration Safety and Innovation Act. Raulerson has been particularly involved with FDA's efforts to incentivize and appropriately regulate abuse-deterrent formulations of opioids and safety-enhancing packaging and disposal technologies for drugs of abuse. He has also helped develop and implement FDA's approach toward the labeling and non-proprietary naming of biosimilar products. Raulerson earned his J.D. at the University of Michigan Law School.

James Shamp is an entrepreneur, technologist, and business executive with more than 18 years of experience in the design, development, operation, and assessment of risk evaluation and mitigation strategy and risk management programs. He is currently the vice president of data intelligence and program analytics at United BioSource, LLC (UBC). He was the founder and former president of J Shamp Consulting LLC. He is the former managing partner of Examoto LLC, which was acquired by UBC. Examoto, a UBC company, focuses on innovation, with the goal of maximizing the benefits and safe use of prescription drugs while reducing the burden to patients, health care providers, and the health care delivery system.

Susan Sherman, Ph.D., M.P.H., is a professor in the Department of Health, Behavior and Society at the Johns Hopkins Bloomberg School of Public Health who focuses on improving the health of marginalized populations, particularly that of drug users and sex workers. She is interested in the structural drivers of health and risk in the conduct of both observational and intervention research. She has more than 17 years of experience in developing and evaluating HIV prevention, peer-outreach, behavioral, and microenterprise interventions in Baltimore, Pakistan, Thailand, and

India. She is the co-director of the Baltimore HIV Collaboratory and a part of the Executive Leadership Committee of the Johns Hopkins Center for AIDS Research. She co-leads the Addiction and Overdose workgroup of the Bloomberg American Health Initiative. She is the principal investigator of a study that examines the role of the police on the sexually transmitted infection/HIV risk environment of street-based sex workers and includes the first cohort of sex workers in the United States. She is also evaluating an innovative prebooking diversion program for low-level drug offenders. She has a new study that focuses on the effects of a structural-level intervention with sex workers in Baltimore and which will create a full service drop-in center for them in that city. She serves on several Baltimore City and state advisory commissions on syringe exchange and overdose prevention initiatives. She is the board secretary of the National Harm Reduction Coalition. Dr. Sherman earned her M.P.H. from the University of North Carolina at Chapel Hill and her Ph.D. from the Johns Hopkins Bloomberg School of Public Health.

Margaret Shield, Ph.D., is a public health and environmental health consultant based in Seattle. She combines a background as a health sciences researcher with more than 18 years of experience working on legislative and regulatory initiatives at the local, state, and national levels. Since 2008, Dr. Shield has been working on solutions for safe, convenient, and environmentally sound disposal of unwanted and expired medications from residents to reduce misuse, diversion, poisonings, and pollution. She has operational and policy experience with residential drug take-back programs, pharmaceutical waste regulation, and drug stewardship policies at the national, state, and local levels. She began this work as a policy staff member for King County, Washington's Local Hazardous Waste Management Program as it worked with partners to develop a secure and convenient pharmacy-based medicine return program. These model protocols informed development of the Drug Enforcement Administration's 2014 rule on controlled substances disposal. She led policy staff for the King County Board of Health's process to pass a 2013 county-wide secure medicine return regulation and subsequently consulted for local health agencies in four other counties that also enacted local pharmaceutical stewardship ordinances. She was a leader in passing the WA Secure Drug Take-Back Act in 2018, the first law in the nation requiring the pharmaceutical industry to provide this critical service. She consulted for the Oregon Department of Environmental Quality on its similar 2019 safe drug disposal law. She researched two reports for the San Francisco Department of the Environment, examining medicine disposal products and whether available information supports their performance claims. Dr. Shield earned her Ph.D. at the University of Washington.

Marta Sokolowska, Ph.D., is the deputy center director for substance use and behavioral health in the Food and Drug Administration's (FDA's) Center for Drug Evaluation and Research (CDER). She serves as the center's executive-level leader responsible for advancing FDA's public health response to the non-medical use of substances with abuse potential. With expertise in science-based assessment and management of drug abuse risks, Dr. Sokolowska advises senior FDA officials on shaping scientific and policy interventions and executing strategies pertaining to the use of controlled substances and behavioral health programs. Dr. Sokolowska joined CDER in 2018 as associate director for controlled substances in the Office of the Center Director. In 2020, she began leading the Controlled Substances Program, which comprises the Controlled Substance Staff (CSS) and the Controlled Substances Initiatives group. CSS provides consultation throughout FDA on evaluation of abuse potential of drugs and advises on all matters related to domestic and international drug scheduling. The strategy group pursues activities and policies to identify, mitigate, and manage emerging issues with controlled substances to minimize risks associated with problematic use while enabling appropriate access to these products for medical use. Prior to joining FDA, Dr. Sokolowska held senior clinical and medical leadership roles in the pharmaceutical industry. She earned her doctoral degree in psychology from McMaster University in Canada.

CDR Andrea Tsatoke, M.P.H., is currently the Indian Health Service (IHS) headquarters injury prevention specialist, focusing on the Tribal Injury Prevention Cooperative Agreement Program (TIPCAP). Commander (CDR) Tsatoke previously served for 6 years in the IHS Phoenix Area Division of Environmental Health Services as the district injury prevention coordinator. She managed the Eastern Arizona Injury Prevention Program, assisting Tribal communities by focusing on the injuries affecting its ~50,000 service population. CDR Tsatoke's career also included IHS assignments in Nevada, California, Alaska, and North Dakota. She has a B.S. in environmental health from Illinois State University and a master's in public health leadership from the University of North Carolina at Chapel Hill. She is also a graduate of the IHS Injury Prevention Fellowship.